Perinatal Risk and Infant Development

Perinatal Risk and Infant Development

ASSESSMENT AND PREDICTION

VICTORIA J. MOLFESE
Southern Illinois University at Carbondale

Foreword by Linda S. Siegel

THE GUILFORD PRESS
New York London

A Division of Guilford Publications, Inc.
72 Spring Street, New York, NY 10012

Printed in the United States of America

Last digit is print number: 9 8 7 6 5 4 3 2 1

Library of Congress Cataloging-in-Publication Data

Molfese, Victoria J.
Perinatal risk and infant development: Assessment and prediction / Victoria J. Molfese.
p. cm.
Bibliography: p.
Includes index.
ISBN 0-89862-728-1
1. Pregnancy, Complications of. 2. Infants (Newborn)—Health risk assessment. I. Title.
[DNLM: 1. Pregnancy Complications. 2. Pregnancy Outcome. 3. Prenatal Diagnosis. 4. Risk Factors. WQ 209 M719a]
RG572.M63 1989
618.3—dc19
DNLM/DLC
for Library of Congress 88-24326
CIP

For the inspiration—

A. VICTORIA JONES
JAMES F. JONES

DENNIS L. MOLFESE
DAVID L. MOLFESE
PETER J. MOLFESE

Foreword

Many infants and their mothers experience difficulties during pregnancy, labor, delivery, and the period immediately after birth. If there was a reliable way to decide who these mothers and infants were, then it might be possible to prevent problems from developing or becoming more serious. Screening for possible prenatal and perinatal problems and outcomes is obviously an important public health issue. One way of accomplishing this task is with a risk index.

Victoria Molfese has undertaken the challenging task of examining scales that are designed to evaluate the degree of risk associated with prenatal and perinatal conditions. The differences and similarities among the scales are discussed, as is the evidence, or lack thereof, for their reliability and validity. The author has also noted, quite rightly, that often these scales are not really based on empirical evidence by on clinical perceptions, and she offers many insightful comments on these risk indices.

This book is not merely a summary of studies but a careful consideration of a number of critical issues in this area. Often risk indices quantify the risk; that is, they assign a specific score indicating the degree of risk. However, when a decision has to be made about an individual case, such as a medical intervention or providing an infant stimulation program, then we must know whether or not the child is at risk, and so a categorical decision is necessary. Dr. Molfese has considered the risk indices from this important perpective. In this connection, she recognizes the significance of the cutoff scores (i.e., specific scores that define the border between "no risk" and "risk"), crucial for decision making about an individual case.

Dr. Molfese has also emphasized the need to differentiate outcomes when considering risk indices. Difficult pregnancies are different from complicated deliveries, and developmental problems are yet another kind of outcome. The particular variables and the weight given to them in the risk index are a function of a specific outcome, a point often missed in the discussion of risk indices. We also need to give differential weights to various outcomes. Developmental language problems may be of more consequence than delayed motor development or some short-term illnesses in the perinatal period that have no long-term ill effects.

The author recognizes the importance of calculating the sensitivity and specificity of risk indices—how a scale can differentiate risk status from no-risk status, and whether too many infants or mothers are detected as being at risk or too many cases are missed.

She acknowledges that some risk factors may be more important than others and that further study of the validity of these risk scales from this perspective is needed. In this light, the author and her colleagues have conducted some important empirical comparisons of these scales. As she also notes, even if we are successfully able to detect who is at risk, we need to make sure that there are suitable treatments available.

It is very important for any risk model to include a number of factors. Dr. Molfese presents a sophisticated multivariate model of risk, including environmental stresses, personality factors, support systems, and individual biological factors. I am not convinced that a risk index needs to be excessively complex, but it does need to consider a number of biological and environmental factors. In addition, the variables in the risk index need to be easily quantifiable, and it should be feasible to collect the information. Although possibly valuable, it is not really practicable to collect data on personality scales or IQ test scores from large samples.

No risk index can be perfectly accurate. This inaccuracy, even if small, leaves us with the dilemma of errors of prediction and what to do with them. If we identify children as being "not at risk" and the children, in fact, develop a problem, then we have missed an opportunity to possibly prevent the problem through intervention. If we identify children as being "at risk" who would not develop a problem, we have identified too many children and may unnecessarily place those children in some treatment or intervention program and inappropriately "label" them.

If errors have to be made, I favor the route of over-identification, preferring false positives to false negatives. There is some evidence that infant stimulation programs offered to young children with potential problems are effective, and no evidence that they are harmful. If we miss a chance to identify the at-risk child, then a valuable opportunity is lost. The identification of such children needs to be done in a sensitive manner to avoid any possible negative effects of labeling. One alternative is not to have any risk indices and to intervene with all children. This is obviously impractical and a waste of time and money. The richest countries in the world cannot afford it, and, even if they could, they would most likely not choose to spend so much money on children.

This book is a very important first step. The next step should be the consideration of the risk indices that can be used to predict developmental outcome. However, to be useful a risk index must be "simple, reliable, and cost-effective," as Dr. Molfese has stated. I share her optimism that we can develop effective and simple ways to assess children at risk. There is evidence that both risk indices (e.g., studies such as those of Tiffany Field, Craig Ramey, and their associates, and myself) and infant test scores (e.g., those of Sarale Cohen and Arthur Parmelee, Ronald Wilson, and myself) can predict developmental outcome to some extent. Obviously, we still have a long way to go, but the early detection of potential developmental problems will not only save money and mental anguish but provide our children with more satisfying and enriched lives.

LINDA S. SIEGEL
The Ontario Institute for Studies in Education

Preface

Studies of infant and child development have increasingly looked toward multivariate models and theories to help explain and predict the growth of mental, physical, and social abilities at different ages. Many of the newer multivariate theories have evolved largely in response to the compelling case made by Sameroff and Chandler (1975) in statements about their transactional model. According to Sameroff and Chandler, there are wide-ranging and bidirectional effects between the environment and the developing organism that cannot be accounted for by simplistic models. These newer multivariate theories have come to include an increasing number of complex variables such a socioeconomic status, parental education, quality of home environment, parenting sytles, behavioral assessments, and selected details of the mothers' and infants' medical histories. The focus of this book is on the medical conditions that have been examined as possible influences on the present and future developmental status of infants and children.

Medical conditions have been particularly intriguing to researchers within medical and behavioral fields because of the difficulties encountered in identifying the specific medical conditions that give rise to abnormal developments in infancy and childhood. The identification of such medical conditions (called "risk conditions") has been particularly difficult in prospective studies, in which estimates of future developmental status are made from assessments of medical conditions obtained during the prenatal or neonatal period. In comparison, retrospective studies have had somewhat greater successes in tracing abnormal development in infancy and childhood to prenatal and neonatal medical conditions. However, because the pool of medical risk conditions is large and the variety of abnormal developments that researchers are seeking to explain and predict is also large, the links between medical conditions and later developmental status frequently have been only weakly demonstrated.

One approach to using medical risk conditions, which is the focus of this book, involves the use of perinatal risk scales. Research findings have been consistent in supporting hypotheses concerning the importance of events that surround the period of birth (the perinatal period). The perinatal period has been found to influence both the status of the infant during the neonatal period and the mental, physical, and social developments that occur during childhood, and is thus of great interest to researchers and practitioners. There have been many efforts to identify and quantify those medical conditions in the perinatal period found to be the most predictive of later developmental status. Indeed, a number of different perinatal risk scales or, in some instances, informal lists of perinatal risk conditions have been used in both prospective and retrospective research designs.

The purpose of this book is to provide a frame of reference for increasing the understanding of medical risk conditions that occur during the perinatal period and how they can be used in predictive models of infant and child development. The targeted readership of the book includes researchers, practictioners, and students who work with normal and abnormal populations of infants and children. Chapters include information on different approaches to the assessment of perinatal risk conditions (including different types of perinatal risk scales, definitions of perinatal risk, and issues of specificity and sensitivity of risk scores) and how such assessment has been used in research studies. Because the medical terminology used to describe and define scale items is frequently unfamiliar to those outside of the medical professions, a glossary is provided for the medical risk conditions included on the perinatal risk scales discussed in this book.

In large part, the motivation for writing this book came from the difficulties we encountered in trying to understand and utilize medical risk conditions within our research on cognitive development during infancy. Because of the variety of available perinatal risk scales and the lack of comparative data on the scales with respect to their predictive validity for use in cognitive research, it was impossible to justify the use of one scale over another in our work. The hope is that this book will make the choice of approach to perinatal risk assessment easier for future researchers.

There are many people who contributed in very important ways to the writing of this book. Dr. Dennis Molfese, my frequent coauthor and colleague, has played a significant part by maintaining the highest standards for the selection and implementation of the methodologies used in the collection and analysis of two large longitudinal studies. The data from these longitudinal studies, supported by grants from the National Foundation/March of Dimes (12142) and the National Institutes of Health (5R1HD17860), have served in part as the basis for three perinatal risk studies of predictive validity. Ms. Karen Yaple has been responsible for the development of the glossary of medical risk terms and the supervision of medical history and behavioral assessment data archives. In both of these activities, she has shown an inspired level of attention to details. As a friend and colleague she is a treasure. In addition, my other graduate students have contributed to the collection and analysis of data, the evaluation of published literature on perinatal risk assessments, and the discussion of theory and research design that have influenced my thinking on these topics. Dr. Brian Thomson, Dr. Mary Bricker, Dr. Blair Beadnell, Ms. Katie Moirs, and Ms. Leslie Manion have played important roles in the development and execution of our research. Special thanks goes to Dr. Allan Bennett, Dr. William Hamilton, and Dr. Philip Sunshine, my medical consultants and research associates, for their help in expanding our understanding of perinatal risks. Finally, thanks to Mrs. Maxine Pierce and Mrs. Jean Heckle for their help in producing the typed manuscript.

Contents

Perinatal Risk and Infant Development

CHAPTER

1

Introduction

Infant populations have been studied for both the prevalence and the consequences of perinatal morbidity and mortality. Results of these studies have been published in a variety of research, case history, and literature survey reports. In general, reports of these studies have noted that approximately 85% of the cases of perinatal mortality and morbidity can be identified as coming from the approximately 25% of pregnancies that are characterized by complications during the antepartum and/or intrapartum periods, complications that have placed the infants at moderate to high risk for poor perinatal outcomes (Wilson & Schifrin, 1980; Nesbitt & Aubry, 1969; Halliday, Jones, & Jones, 1980). The consequences suffered by infants born to women whose pregnancies are characterized by high-risk complications have been of particular concern. These infants are more likely to die during the perinatal period, and surviving infants are more likely to have multiple problems during the neonatal period that require medical and surgical teatments, special nursing care, and longer hospital stays. In later infancy and in childhood, these infants are more likely to experience complications that are associated with the neonatal conditions of prematurity, low birthweight, asphyxia, respiratory distress syndrome, and low 1- and 5-minute Apgar scores (Akhtar & Sehgal, 1980; Hobel, Hyvarinen, Okada, & Oh, 1973; Prechtl, 1967; Shapiro, Schlesinger, & Nesbitt, 1968; Sokol, Rosen, Stojkov, & Chik, 1977). Complications such as mental retardation, cerebral palsy, minimal cerebral dysfunctions, seizure disorders, and abnormalities in perceptual and cognitive functioning have frequently been identified. It appears that appropriate therapeutic interventions for reducing fetal and infant morbidity and mortality can be planned and instituted if the conditions that give rise to perinatal risks are identified early in pregnancy (Ryan, Sweeney, & Solola, 1980; Simmons, 1978; Sokol, Woolf, Rosen, & Weingarden, 1980). However, there has been considerable debate over how best to screen for perinatal risk conditions so that both outcome and cost-effectiveness are maximized.

In addition to clinical applications, screening for perinatal risk conditions has also become important to researchers studying infant and child development. These researchers have been interested in developing objective screening methods for quantifying the risk-producing conditions in pregnancy, labor, and delivery. Quantifying the risk conditions permits them to be used in statistical models designed to predict behaviors in infancy and childhood. These objective methods have typically involved procedures in which specific perinatal complications are identified and scores are assigned to those complications. The numerical scores assigned to complications vary in magnitude, to reflect the differing levels of risk for poor developmental consequences during infancy and childhood. However, the specific complications that are assessed by the various objective methods vary widely, and there seems to be little agreement as to how the complications should best be assessed. In addition, perinatal risk scores have often been found to be only weak predictors of behaviors in infancy and later childhood. The weak contribution of perinatal risk scores seems to be due more to the limited types of complications included on assessment scales and to deficiencies in the procedures used to assign scores to perinatal risks than to the unimportance of perinatal risks *per se*.

The problems involved in identifying perinatal conditions that produce risks of morbidity and mortality can be illustrated in the following descriptions of two women: The first woman has the following characteristics: age = 31 years, marital status = single, weight at delivery = 178 pounds, parity = 7, acute/chronic diseases in pregnancy = urinary tract infection, time since last pregnancy = 7 years, number of prenatal visits = 3, smoking = 1 to 2 packs per day, nutritional status = poor to fair. The second woman is characterized by the following: age

= 25 years, marital status = married, weight at delivery = 184 pounds, parity = 0, acute/chronic diseases in pregnancy = hydrocephalus with shunt, number of prenatal visits = 10, smoking = no, nutritional status = excellent.

From these descriptions, how would one evaluate these women for their level of perinatal risk ("high" vs. "medium" vs. "low")? What conditions would be used as the basis by which one could differentiate between the two women in terms of the relative levels of risk each woman has? Clearly, there are serious conditions that characterize both women. Yet, which conditions would place these women at greatest risk? Evaluations of perinatal conditions have commonly been made on the basis of the clinical judgment of physicians. However, initial evaluations in early pregnancy could also be rendered through the utilization of a screening system that would serve to alert medical personnel to the presence of certain targeted high-risk conditions. Lesinksi (1975) notes that the ideal screening system should be simple, reliable, and easy to apply. Although there has been little disagreement that evaluations for perinatal risk should ideally be made using a combination of clinical judgment and a risk scoring system, there has been considerable disagreement on how best to implement a system of perinatal risk scoring that is both accurate and effective.

Standardized methods for assessing perinatal data for poor pregnancy outcome have been recommended as one means of implementing such a scoring system (Hobel, 1978). These assessment methods have been recommended because they can be useful in both clinical and research applications in several ways. Medical records contain a vast amount of diverse perinatal information, including medical history; socioeconomic status; ongoing records of all patient care and treatment provided during pregnancy, including the results of physical examinations, laboratory work, and prognoses; detailed time sheets recording labor progress, procedures, and medications administered during labor; fetal monitoring tracings and interpretations; procedures, medications, and outcome of the delivery process; and a variety of detailed measures pertaining to the postnatal status of the mother and infant. This mass of information contained in medical records can be translated into a condensed, yet comprehensive, record consisting of specific perinatal conditions that are known or thought to produce poor perinatal outcomes.

Ideally, the use of these condensed records can maximize the accurate assessment of medical information by physicians and researchers while minimizing errors due to oversight. The increase in accuracy can occur because the perinatal conditions contained in the condensed records would be those that have been evaluated by clinicians and researchers because of their potential for producing poor maternal and infant outcomes. The conditions of importance are highlighted by their inclusion on the condensed record and therefore stand out against the masses of other information in the medical record. By assigning scores to these important or critical conditions according to the severity of the poor outcomes, the perinatal risks associated with these conditions can be quantified. For example, early vaginal bleeding has been found to be related to a higher incidence of infant complications (e.g., low birthweight, low gestational age, perinatal death, asphyxia, breech delivery, placental infarcts, and small-for-gestational-age infants) (Batzofin, Fielding, & Friedman, 1984; Funderburk, Guthrie, & Meldrum, 1980). Obesity in pregnancy, on the other hand, is associated with complications in pregnancy (e.g., hypertension, inadequate pregnancy weight gain, diabetes, repeat cesarean section), but complications during labor and the postnatal status of the infant have not been found to be significantly different from those associated with women who are not obese (Gross, Sokol, & King, 1980). By giving a larger score to early vaginal bleeding than to obesity, the level of patient risk for poor infant outcomes due to these factors would be differentially quantified. If level of patient risk for complications of pregnancy and labor were targeted conditions, then obesity would be given a larger score than early vaginal bleeding. Thus, specific types of perinatal risks could be reflected in the scores assigned to the perinatal conditions.

Clinicians and researchers have responded to the call for standardized methods of assessing conditions that produce perinatal risk by proposing a variety of screening scales. All of these screening scales have been developed for particular obstetric populations for the purpose of reducing maternal and infant morbidity and mortality through the early and accurate identification of risk conditions. As commonly used, "morbidity" refers to incidences of injury and pathology and to various types of abnormalities and anomalies (e.g., hemorrhaging and fever in postpartum women, and meconium aspiration and prematurity in neonates). "Mortality" refers to instances of maternal and infant deaths, including miscarriages and stillbirths. Conditions affecting both morbidity and mortality as outcomes are included in the perinatal risk scales that are described in this chapter and in subsequent chapters.

TYPES OF PERINATAL RISK SCALES

A number of perinatal risk scales have been developed for use in screening pregnant women, and some for also screening neonates for problems that might arise during later developmental periods as a result of antepartum and intrapartum problems. These perinatal risk scales contain items related to a variety of complications that can arise during pregnancy, labor and delivery, or the postnatal period. Prechtl's (1968) definition of "complications" seems to best summarize the assumptions underlying these scales. According to Prechtl, an obstetric complication is "any factor or group of factors in the pre- or perinatal environment which increases the risk of fetal mortality. These will be symptoms of maternal disease during pregnancy, signs of fetal distress and mechanical intervention in the delivery. Few of these factors are independent of each other and many are causally related" (p. 20).

The specific complications that are included on each scale vary as a result of differences in the perceptions of the clinicians and reseachers who developed the scales regarding what risks should be screened and how the risks should be evaluated. Typically, the specific complications included on a scale are based on the personal experience of the scale developer, are drawn from other perinatal risk scales, or are selected on the basis of research findings. These complications may pertain to the antepartum period (the period prior to birth), the intrapartum period (the period during labor and delivery), both the antepartum and intrapartum periods, or the postpartum period.

Antepartum Risk Scales

For many scale developers, the antepartum period is seen as the optimal time for screening patients for perinatal risk (Goodwin, Dunne, & Thomas, 1969; Coopland *et al.,* 1977). For many developers, early screening permits existing antepartum complications to be identified and remedied before the onset of additional complications that might arise during labor and delivery. Many developers also see the antepartum period as more amenable to screening, since the scale can be administered during the first antepartum visit and at additional times during pregnancy as needed. Indeed, patients considered "high risk" based on the complications noted during the screening of antepartum events can receive prenatal care offering a variety of medical interventions for treatable complications. These interventions can reduce the actual complications during pregnancy, labor, and delivery and can also lower the postpartum risks. Such intervention effects based on antepartum screening have been reported for a variety of different types of patients by several investigators (e.g., Nesbitt & Aubry, 1971; Ryan *et al.,* 1980).

Examples of two scales that screen for antepartum risks only are shown in Tables 1-1 and 1-2. The Prenatal High-Risk Scoring Form (Coopland *et al.,* 1977) contains three categories of items: reproductive history, associated conditions, and present pregnancy. Each item has an assigned risk score ranging from 0 to 3; scores for all items can be totaled to produce a summary score. On this scale, summary scores can be obtained for the first prenatal visit and again at 36 weeks. Assignment to a "low-risk," "high-risk," or "extreme-risk" category can be made using the risk point cutoffs provided by the scale developers.

A second scale that screens only for antepartum risks is the Antepartum Fetal Risk Scale (Goodwin *et al.,* 1969). The items

Table 1-1. Coopland, Peddle, Baskett, Rollwagen, Simpson, and Parker's (1977) Prenatal High-Risk Scoring Form

Score each question as indicated. Total each category score at 1st visit. Repeat at 36 weeks.

I. Reproductive history		II. Associated conditions		III. Present pregnancy	
Age <16	= 1	Previous gynecological surgery	= 1	Bleeding	
16–35	= 0	Chronic renal disease	= 2	< 20 wk	= 1
>35	= 2	Gestational diabetes	= 1	> 20 wk	= 3
Parity 0	= 1	Diabetes mellitus	= 3	Anemia < 10 gm %	= 1
1–4	= 0	Cardiac disease	= 3	Prolonged pregnancy (42 weeks)	= 1
5+	= 2	Other medical disorders (chronic bronchitis,		Hypertension	= 2
Past OB history		lupus, etc.)		Premature rupture of membranes	= 2
Habitual abortion/infertility	= 1	Score according to severity		Polyhydramnios	= 2
PPH/manual removal	= 1	(1 to 3)	= __	Small for dates	= 3
Baby >9 lb (4,082 gm)	= 1			Multiple pregnancy	
Baby <5½ lb (2,500 gm)	= 1			Breech	= 3
PET/hypertension	= 1			Malpresentation	
Previous cesarean	= 2			Rh isoimmunization	= 3
Stillbirth or neonatal death	= 3				
Prolonged labor or difficult delivery	= 1				
Category score	____+	Category score	____+	Category score	____

Total risk score 1st visit = ____ Total at 36 weeks = ____

(Record scores in box on prenatal sheet.)

Note: Low risk = 0–2
High risk = 3–6
Extreme risk = 7 >

Note. From "A Simplified Antepartum High-Risk Pregnancy Scoring Form: Statistical Analysis of 5459 Cases" by A. T. Coopland, L. J. Peddle, T. F. Baskett, R. Rollwagen, A. Simpson, and E. Parker, 1977. *Canadian Medical Association Journal, 116*, p. 1000. Copyright 1977 by the Canadian Medical Association. Reprinted by permission.

TABLE 1-2. Goodwin, Dunne, and Thomas's (1969) Antepartum Fetal Risk Score

Baseline data		Obstetric history	
Age 35+	1	Abortion	
Age 40+	2	Stillbirth	
Para 0	1	Neonatal death	
Para 6+	2	Surviving premature infant	
Interval < 2 yr	1	Antepartum hemmorrhage	
Obesity (200 lb +; 90 kg+)	1	Toxemia	
Diabetes B, C, D	2	Difficult midforceps delivery	
F	3	Cesarean section	
Chronic renal disease	1	Major congenital anomaly	
With diminished renal function	3	Baby 10 lb+ (or 4.5kg+)	
With increased blood urea nitrogen	3		
		One instance of above	1
Hypertension (pre-existing)		Two or more instances in different pregnancies	2
$\frac{140+}{90+}$ 1 $\frac{160+}{110+}$	2	Rh isoimmunized mother	
		+ Homozygous father	2
		+ History of erythroblastosis	3

Score (circle one) 0 1 2 3

Present pregnancy			
Bleeding, early (<20 wk)		Toxemia I	1
Alone 1		Toxemia II	3
With pain 2		Eclampsia II	3
Bleeding, late (>20 wk)		Hydramnios (single fetus)	3
Ceased	1	Multiple pregnancy	2
Continues	2		
With pain	3	Abnormal glucose tolerance	1
With hypotension	3	Decreasing insulin requirement	3
		Maternal acidosis	3
Spontaneous premature rupture of membranes	1	Maternal pyrexia	1
Latent period 24 hr+	2	Pyrexia + fetal heart rate > 160	2
Anemia <10 gm Hb	1	Rh negative	
< 8 gm Hb	2	With rising titer	2
No prenatal care	2	With amniotic fluid Liley zone III	3
< 3 prenatal visits	1		

Score (circle one) 0 1 2 3

(continued)

TABLE 1-2. (*Continued*)

Gestational age			
28 wk or under	4	37 wk or under	1
32 wk or under	3	42 wk or under	1
35 wk or under	2	43 wk or under	2
Score (circle one)	0 1 2 3		

Note. From "Antepartum Identification of the Fetus at Risk" by J. W. Goodwin, J. T. Dunne, and B. W. Thomas, 1969. *Canadian Medical Association Journal, 101,* p. 59. Copyright 1969 by the Canadian Medical Association. Reprinted by permission.

on this scale are divided into three categories: baseline and obstetrical history, present pregnancy, and gestational age. Each item has an assigned risk score ranging from 1 to 3. Summary scores ranging from 0 to 4 points can be given for each of the three categories.

These antepartum scales are similar to each other and to other antepartum scales in a number of respects. Antepartum scales typically include items designed to give baseline data (e.g., maternal age, parity, reproductive history, and preexisting medical complications). In addition, these scales contain items that pertain to a variety of specific complications that may have developed during the current pregnancy. Some scales also include items pertaining to socioeconomic status (e.g., marital status, education, income) and race.

Recent reports have indicated that antepartum screening alone does not produce the hoped-for reduction in perinatal morbidity and mortality. Wilson and Schifrin (1980) reviewed the reported incidents of morbidity and mortality in five studies. As shown in Table 1-3, groups that were identified as "low risk" during the antepartum period were found to have about the same incidence of perinatal morbidity and mortality as did groups identified as "high risk." Both the "low-risk" and the "high-risk" groups contributed about 50% of the perinatal morbidity and mortality.

This report on the inadequacy of screening only during the antepartum period was confirmed in two separate studies. In one study (Rosenberg, Albertsen, Jones, & Roberts, 1981), data were obtained on 240,000 pregnancies that had no antepartum complications. However, in 21% of these pregnan-

TABLE 1-3. Wilson and Schifrin's (1980) Risk Classification Based on Various Social, Demographic, and Historic Factors Related to Outcome

Author	Risk classification	Patients: Number	Patients: Percent	Contribution to perinatal mortality and morbidity	
Hobel (1975);	Antepartum low risk	962	68	PNM&M	48%
Hobel, Hyvarinen,	Antepartum high risk	455	32	PNM&M	52%
Okada, and Oh (1973)		1,417	100		
Donahue and Wan	3 low-risk quartiles		75	PNM	56%
(1975)	1 high-risk quartile		25	PNM	43%
			100		
Goodwin, Dunne,	2 low-risk groups	248	62	PNM	39%
and Thomas (1969)	3 high-risk groups	148	38	PNM	61%
		396	100		
Nesbitt and Aubry	Low and	699	64	PNM&M	53%
(1969)	moderate risk	388	36	PNM&M	47%
	High risk	1,087	100		
Feldstein and	Low risk (age only)	10,380	61	PNM	53%
Butler (1965)	High risk (age only)	6,603	39	PNM	47%
		16,983	100		
Totals	Low risk	11,358	67	PNM	58%
	High risk (age, parity,	5,625	33	PNM	42%
	class)	16,983	100		

Note. PNM = perinatal mortality; M = morbidity. From "Ideas & Actions: Is Any Pregnancy Low Risk?" by R. W. Wilson and B. S. Schifrin, 1980. *Obstetrics and Gynecology, 55,* p. 654. Copyright 1980 by Elsevier Science Publishing Co. Reprinted by permission of The American College of Obstetricians and Gynecologists.

cies, complications developed later, during labor and delivery. In the second study, Hobel *et al.* (1973) concluded that intrapartum events are more important predictors of perinatal outcomes than are antepartum events (Table 1-4). These authors reported that mothers who scored as "high risk" during the intrapartum period, regardless of the level of their antepartum risk, had a neonatal morbidity rate three to four times higher and a perinatal mortality rate six to ten times higher than they would have had if they had been at "low risk" during the intrapartum period. Further, they noted that about 23% of the women who were evaluated as "low risk" during

TABLE 1-4. Risk Status and Perinatal Outcomes

High-risk status				Neonatal[a]		Perinatal mortality	
Number	Percent	Prenatal period	Intrapartum period	Number	Percent	Number	Rate
340	46	Low risk[b]	Low risk	22	6.5	1	3/7,000
135	18	High risk[b]	Low risk	16	11.8	3	22/1,000
144	20	Low risk	High risk	35	24.3	5	35/1,000
119	16	High risk	High risk	42	35.0	16	145/1,000
738				115		25	34/1,000[c]

Note. From "Prenatal and Intrapartum High-Risk Screening: I. Prediction of the High-Risk Neonate" by C. J. Hobel, M. A. Hyvarinen, D. M. Okada, and W. Oh, 1973. *American Journal of Obstetrics and Gynecology, 117,* p. 5. Copyright 1973 by C. V. Mosby Co. Reprinted by permission.

[a]Neonatal morbidity = score ≥ 10.

[b]Low risk: total score < 10; high risk: > 10.

[c]Overall perinatal mortality rate.

the antepartum period became "high risk" during the intrapartum period. These women accounted for 33% of the cases of perinatal morbidity and mortality, compared to a 40% perinatal morbidity and mortality rate for the women who were "high risk" during the antepartum and intrapartum periods. These data have been used to argue that antepartum risk screening alone is not adequate for effective identification of perinatal morbidity and mortality.

INTRAPARTUM RISK SCALES

As an alternative to screening only during the antepartum period, researchers have proposed adding intrapartum screening, so that complications that arise during labor and delivery can be identified as well. Some of the developers of these intrapartum scales have argued that effective screening of conditions producing perinatal risks can be done during labor, particularly if the screening occurs during the first stage of labor rather than during the shorter second stage. These developers believe that screening early in labor would allow enough time to remedy complications or to institute appropriate management procedures.

One example of an intrapartum screening scale is that which was developed by Morrison, Carter, McNamara, and Cheang (1980). This scale (shown in Table 1-5) consists of 12 items divided into three categories: labor, associated conditions, and miscellaneous. Risk scores range from 1 to 4. In a study of 1,994 pregnant women, 24% were classified as "high risk" during the intrapartum period, using scores of 3 or greater; 72% of the cases of neonatal mortality and neonatal and maternal morbidity occurred in this "high-risk" group, whereas 73% of the normal outcomes occurred in the "low-risk" group.

A second intrapartum screening scale is that of Aubry and Pennington (1973) (see Chapter 2, Table 2-9). This scale was developed to provide a means of separating low- and high-risk obstetric patients beyond that already provided by an antepartum scale (the Nesbitt and Aubry scale [Nesbitt & Aubry, 1969]) currently in place as a screening device. The scale has

TABLE 1-5. Morrison, Carter, McNamara, and Cheang's (1980) Intrapartum Screening Scale

Factor	Score
Labor	
Labor ⩾ 20 hr	2
Slow latent phase progress—<3 cm dilation with contractions for 10 hr	1
Slow active phase progress—"no progress" or <1.5 cm dilation in 2 hr	2
Meconium in first stage—dark, fresh, or heavy	4
Meconium in first stage—light, old staining	1
Associated conditions	
Gestation <34 wk	3
Premature rupture of membranes ⩾ 24 hr	2
Syntocinon induction or augmentation of labor	2
Miscellaneous	
Height: <5 ft 2 in (155 cm)	1
Weight: <100 lb (45 kg) ⩾200 lb (90 kg)	1
Smoking (current): ⩾20 to 25 cigarettes per day	1
Ethnic: North American Indian	1

Note. From "A Simplified Intrapartum Numerical Scoring System" by I. Morrison, L. Carter, S. McNamara, and M. Cheang, 1980. *American Journal of Obstetrics and Gynecology, 138,* p. 176. Copyright 1980 by C. V. Mosby Co. Reprinted by permission.

items representing 14 categories of complications; the risk scores assigned to each item range from 10 to 30 points.

Intrapartum screening scales typically include items pertaining to the length of the first stage of labor, progression of the dilation process, presence of meconium, gestational age, length of time in which the membranes were ruptured, incidence of labor induction or augmentation, and use of drugs and medications. Some scales also include items pertaining to the antepartum characteristics of the patient (e.g., height, weight, race, number of prenatal visits, parity) and some selected antepartum items usually related to risk factors that have been present during the antepartum period.

Some of the intrapartum scales have been used in conjunction with antepartum scales, with a noted increase in correct identification of patients at risk (Aubry & Pennington, 1973; Akhtar & Sehgal, 1980; Morrison *et al.*, 1980). In the Morrison *et al.* (1980) study, the 472 patients who scored as "high risk" during the intrapartum period accounted for 31% of the cases of morbidity. However, when antepartum scores were included, those patients with high antepartum and intrapartum risk accounted for 71% of the morbidity cases. Aubry and Pennington (1973) studied the outcomes of the pregnancies of 450 women. "Negative perinatal outcomes" were defined as instances of prematurity, low birthweight infants, neonatal depression, and/or respiratory distress syndrome. Based on antepartum scores, twice as many of the high-risk women had negative perinatal outcomes as the low-risk women. When intrapartum scores were added, the greatest proportion of negative perinatal outcomes was found to come from the sample of women who obtained high-risk scores on both the antepartum and the intrapartum scales. Improvements in predictions such as these have encouraged scale developers to include complications pertaining to more than one perinatal period.

Antepartum, Intrapartum, and Postpartum Risk Scales

The most frequently used type of perinatal risk scale contains items pertaining to the antepartum, intrapartum, and postpartum periods. This book will focus on scales of this type because these are the scales that are particularly suitable for use in predictive models of infant outcome and child development. These scales have several advantages over other types of scales, but the main advantage is the addition of the postpartum items. Recognition of the different impacts of antepartum and intrapartum risks on outcome has resulted in the development of screening scales that make it possible to assess the impact of these risks on specific aspects of the postnatal status of the mother and the infant. Most frequently, the postpartum items pertain exclusively to the postnatal status of the neonate; because of the focus of this book, only scales of this type will be described.

Typically, the neonatal items pertain to complications involving birthweight, gestational age, heart rate during labor or postnatally, umbilical cord problems, the onset of respiration, and Apgar scores (Apgar, 1953). The most extensive group of neonatal items is contained on the High-Risk Pregnancy Screening System developed by Hobel *et al.* (1973) (see Chapter 2, Table 2-3). This scale includes 35 neonatal items covering categories of respiratory problems, metabolic disorders, cardiac abnormalities, hematologic problems, central nervous system disorders, and general disorders.

Interestingly, the proportion of items on the Hobel *et al.* scale devoted to screening postpartum status is smaller (28%) than the proportion of antepartum (40%) or intrapartum items (32%). This difference in proportion is similar to that found in other perinatal risk scales, in which approximately 12% to 30% of the items pertain to postpartum complications, compared to 22% to 60% for antepartum items and 28% to 48% for intrapartum items. This smaller proportion of postpartum items reflects the orientation of these scales toward pregnancy, labor, and the birth process rather than toward the later functioning of the neonate, although screening for morbidity and mortality of both mother and infant is the ultimate goal of these scales. Researchers are hoping that the scales can be usefully extended beyond the labor and delivery process, toward predicting the later functioning of the neonate and the infant.

DEFINITIONS OF RISK

The complications represented by the scale items are nearly always accompanied by some defining characteristics or definitions by which risk is assessed. In some cases, these characteristics are quite specific. For example, the defining characteristic for maternal age that occurs on various scales usually includes a minimum–maximum age range. On some scales, for example, women who are under 15 years of age or over 35 years are considered to be "at risk" for perinatal complications; women who lie within the minimum–maximum range are not "at risk" on those scales. In many cases, the defining characteristics for a given complication differ from one scale to another. For example, the definitions of risk associated with premature rupture of membranes that are found on several different scales include "present," no time limit specified; "present for over 6 hours"; and "present for over 12 hours." Sometimes, no defining characteristics are given, but the presence or diagnosis of a specific type of condition is used as the definition. For example, "gestational diabetes," "polyhydramnios," and "Rh isoimmunized" are often listed without specific definitions. If the patient has the condition or fits the defining characteristic, then the associated risk score is assigned; if not, no risk score is assigned.

A glossary of antepartum, intrapartum, and neonatal conditions that are frequently included on perinatal risk screening scales is provided at the end of this book. The defining characteristics often associated with each condition are given, along with information on how the condition is uniquely defined on some perinatal risk scales. Although occasionally there are wide variations across scales in the specific defining characteristics for a particular condition, it is important to have information on how such a condition generally is defined. From that basis, the constraints imposed on the condition by the defining characteristics used by a particular scale can be accommodated.

The wide differences in the defining characteristics used for specific perinatal conditions are of importance when considering perinatal risk scales as screening devices. For example, consider the minimum–maximum maternal age range used on perinatal risk scales. On these scales, the cutoff for the minimum age varies from under 15 years to under 18 years; the cutoff for the maximum age may be over 30 years, 35 years, or over 35 years. Depending on the patient's age and on the defining characteristics used by the scales, the patient might be considered at risk on one perinatal scale but not on another.

In an effort to determine what effects the use of different defining characteristics for specific complications would have on subjects' risk scores, Molfese, Thomson, and Bennett (1985) obtained risk scores for a group of subjects on five different perinatal risk scales. Chi-square analyses were conducted on pairwise comparisons of scale items with risk and no-risk groupings of the subjects. These analyses revealed that in most cases, the defining characteristics were similar enough that the subjects' assignments to the risk or no-risk categories did not differ significantly across scales. Indeed, the subjects' assignments to risk categories were highly similar in most cases. However, there were instances in which the number of subjects considered to be "at risk" based on the presence of a specific complication differed across the scales as a result of differences in the specific criteria used to define risk. The analyses showed significant differences between risk and no-risk category assignments in 31% (or 27 of 88) of the possible comparisons of scale items within the antepartum categories, compared to 11% (or 8 of 71) of the possible pairwise comparisons of scale items within the intrapartum categories. Thus the accuracy of the risk predictions made by each of the five scales would be expected to vary for subjects, depending on the defining characteristics used with each complication.

SCORING

All perinatal risk scales assign a score to each condition contained on the scale. The scores are used to calculate a total risk score and, on most scales, separate antepartum, intrapartum, and postpartum risk scores. These scores, in turn, are used as raw scores to represent a continuum of risk or are converted into categories, such as "high risk," "moderate risk," and "low risk." Interestingly, on most scales, the scores assigned to the conditions and the scores used to assign subjects to risk categories are based on the professional judgment of the scale developers as to how important a specific condition or point total is in determining poor perinatal outcomes. Rarely are scores based on empirical evidence, such as studies of their predictive validity. There have been few published criticisms of the process by which scores are assigned to scale conditions, which is surprising, because the scores vary considerably in the magnitude of the numerical penalties assigned. Most scales assign risk points within a relatively restricted range (e.g., from 0 to 4 points). However, some scales range from 0 to 30 points (Nesbitt & Aubry, 1969; Aubry & Pennington, 1973), one scale is based on exact risk probabilities and utilizes penalties ranging from 1.3 to 40.7 (Brazie, Searls, & Lubchenco's scale, cited in Lubchenco, 1976, p. 120), and some scales use a simple "present = 1" or "absent = 0" system (Littman & Parmelee, 1978).

The use, by various scales, of different magnitudes of scores for similar conditions does not usually present problems when only a single scale is used in evaluating perinatal risk. Problems can arise, though, when several scales that differ in the magnitude of scores assigned to similar conditions are used to assess perinatal risk. In a study that examined the risk points assigned to a variety of antepartum and intrapartum items taken from five perinatal risk scales, it was found that the scales frequently differed in terms of the items that were assigned maximum risk points (Molfese *et al.,* 1985). For example, on one scale, "multiple pregnancy" (e.g., twins, triplets) was scored as "high risk" and received the maximum number of points possible on that scale, whereas on the other four scales, it received minimal points and was scored as "low risk." Similar inconsistencies existed for many of the other items. These differences in the magnitude of penalties assigned to similar conditions can produce instances in which point totals would indicate that a subject is "at risk" on one scale but not on another scale. Clearly, this brings into question the validity of the scales for accurately predicting perinatal risk.

Problems have also arisen with regard to how the scores

are utilized. Scores have often been used as the basis for assigning patients to "low-risk," "moderate-risk," and "high-risk" categories. Hobel *et al.* (1973) have found that using risk categories as data for predicting perinatal outcomes does not produce the same results as those obtained when using actual risk scores. These researchers compared the accuracy of actual risk scores versus dichotomized (e.g., "at risk" vs. "not at risk") risk scores in predicting neonatal days in the hospital. Although both actual scores and dichotomized scores were found to be predictive of hospital stay, actual scores were reported to be the more accurate predictors.

Problems have also been reported when total risk scores rather than scores for specific complications are used as the data in predictive studies. Coplan (1980) has noted that the use of total risk scores does not permit one to examine the relationship between specific complications and specific perinatal outcomes. Thus there may not be significant correlations between total risk scores and perinatal outcomes, but such correlations may exist between specific complications and specific perinatal outcomes. Correlations of the latter type are rarely examined in research studies, with total risk score being used almost exclusively. However, the use of specific complications, particularly groups of co-occurring complications, could yield useful information concerning the types of outcomes likely to result. When they have been reported in studies, the correlations produced between single complications and single outcome measures have been low and frequently not significant, but correlations between co-occurring complications and outcome measures have been largely unexplored. It remains the task of future research, utilizing large samples of subjects, to explore the usefulness of single complications and groups of co-occurring complications for predicting perinatal outcomes.

The use of total risk scores has also been criticized by Strobino and Baruffi (1984), in an article in which they evaluate the use of the Hobel *et al.* (1973) neonatal risk scale. These authors compared the results produced by using total risk scores versus those produced by using a count of the number of risk items (complications). In general, the results produced by both methods were similar. However, the number of risk items proved to be significantly related to a negative binomial distribution, which the authors describe as an indication of the extent to which the results are due to a combination of random factors plus inherent characteristics of the subjects. The authors have also recommended that the number of risk items be used as the risk score rather than total risk points, since the former is easier to calculate. The predictive validity of number of risk items for perinatal risk scales has not been reported in the literature but is discussed as part of the research findings of Molfese *et al.* (1985) reported in Chapter 3.

QUESTIONS OF SCALE VALIDITY

Many studies have addressed issues related to the validity of perinatal risk scales in predicting the incidence of maternal and infant morbidity and mortality. The majority of these studies have focused on measures of infant status as the criteria for evaluating the perinatal risk scores. Typically, these studies have examined whether infant status was affected by events that occurred during pregnancy, labor, and/or delivery. Studies of this type can be classified into three groups. The first group has assessed scores derived from perinatal risk scales as predictors of clinically and medically relevant infant outcome measures (e.g., Apgar scores, birthweight, gestational age, infection, birth injuries, neurological abnormalities, respiratory distress, specific physiologic measures, days in the hospital, mortality). Examples of studies in this group are those by Aubry and Pennington (1973); Dixon, Tronick, Keefer, and Brazelton, 1982; Hobel *et al.* (1973); Littman and Parmelee (1978); Prechtl (1967, 1968); Sokol *et al.* (1980); and Zax, Sameroff, and Babigian (1977). Studies in the second group have focused on the ability of perinatal risk scores to predict behavioral measures obtained during the neonatal period (e.g., performance on the Brazelton Neonatal Assessment Scale [Brazelton, 1973], sleep states, cardiac responsivity, visual perception). Examples of studies in this group are those by Lester, Emory, Hoffman, and Eitzman (1976); Rose, Schmidt, Riese, and Bridges (1980); Sepkoski, Coll, and Lester (1977, 1982);

and Werner, Bartlett, and Siqueland (1982). The third group of studies has looked at the ability of perinatal risk scores to predict behavioral measures obtained in later infancy and during childhood (e.g., performance on intelligence tests, language development, developmental stages). Examples of studies in this group are those by Beckwith and Cohen (1980); Bee *et al.* (1982); Broman, Nichols, and Kennedy, (1975); Caputo, Goldstein, and Taub (1981); Cohen and Beckwith (1979); Field *et al.* (1978); Goldstein, Caputo, and Taub (1976); Littman and Parmelee (1978); Sameroff (1979); and Sigman, Cohen, and Forsythe (1981).

Although these studies have provided a wealth of information on the validity of perinatal risk scales and scores, they do have shortcomings. Typically, these studies have included only one scale or only a few risk variables for use in determining the perinatal risk scores. Thus it is hard to evaluate how the predictive accuracy of the scale used in one study compares with that of a different scale used in another study. The perinatal risk scores have also been used in some studies only as subject classification variables (or to provide descriptive information for the subject sample) rather than as dependent variables. Thus there are often no direct statistical assessments of how well perinatal risk scores predict the outcome measures. Those studies that do report such direct assessments usually have found low, but significant, correlations (range = .23 to .48) between perinatal risk scores and a variety of outcome measures obtained during the neonatal period. However, attempts to predict, from perinatal risk scores, outcome measures obtained in later infancy and during childhood have not been as successful. In these latter studies, the correlations are often low and not significant. However, though the magnitude of the correlations is low, it is clear that infants whose status at birth is poor (e.g., low-birthweight infants with various subsequent complications) and who show abnormal development in later infancy can be identified more often than infants without complications as having had a high number of perinatal risk factors. Thus the scales using antepartum and intrapartum risk scores seem to be in need of refinements that will increase the accuracy of predicting outcome measures obtained during later infancy and childhood.

Another issue concerning validity was raised in a recent article by Baruffi, Strobino, and Dellinger (1984). These researchers questioned the validity of perinatal risk scales when used with populations other than those from which they were originally developed. They found that two populations of pregnant women with similar socioeconomic characteristics differed significantly in the distribution of specific perinatal risk items despite efforts to control for the presence of unique risk characteristics in each population. They also found that the accuracy of predicting infant morbidity varied, depending on the definition used to score a patient as "high risk" (e.g., 10 points or more, 15 points or more, or 20 points or more). Cutoff scores useful in one population for classifying patients as "high risk" and for predicting infant morbidity were not necessarily useful for the second population. In addition, comparisons of the predictive validity of perinatal risk scales do not typically include women sampled from more than one population.

Other researchers (Roux, 1976) have suggested that it might be necessary to modify items on a scale in order to adapt that scale to the particular perinatal risk characteristics found in a specific obstetric population. Modifications might involve expanding a scale to include more items pertaining to the antepartum or intrapartum complications that typify a given population or selecting items representing risk factors predictive of the specific types of poor outcomes that occur most frequently in a given population. To date, these potential improvements in scales have not been studied empirically using more than one perinatal risk scale. It needs to be demonstrated that more accurate predictions can be made if patients are screened for perinatal risk by scales that are better suited to the characteristics of the population within which these patients fall.

SENSITIVITY AND SPECIFICITY

Another issue regarding the validity of perinatal risk scales is their ability to accurately classify individuals who are at risk and those who are not. Ideally, perinatal risk scales should identify as being "at risk" only those individuals who will in fact experience perinatal problems if they do not receive remedial treatment and/or those who will remain "at risk" even with remedial treatment. Individuals who are *not* at risk should not be identified by the scale as being at risk. Two concepts that are relevant to a discussion of classification accuracy are sensitivity and specificity. "Sensitivity" refers to the proportion of "at risk" individuals correctly identified by scores on a perinatal risk scale; it indicates the degree to which the "true positives" ("positive" indicating the presence of the negative or abnormal condition) in a sample are identified. In contrast, "specificity" refers to the proportion of normal individuals correctly identified by scores on a perinatal risk scale; it indicates the degree to which "true negatives" ("negative" indicating the absence of the negative condition) are identified.

The sensitivity rate of perinatal risk scores is usually the major focus of scale developers. However, this rate is rarely 100%. Thus, when scores are used to categorize individuals as "normal" or "abnormal," they usually have to be set at a level at which sensitivity is maximized and specificity minimized. If the scores are set too high, the number of individuals identified as being "at risk" might be too small to include all of those who are in fact "at risk." If the scores are set too low, the scale would identify not only many of the individuals "at risk" but also many of the individuals who are in fact not "at risk." In the former case, both outcome effectiveness and cost-effectiveness are minimal because many individuals who are "at risk" are not being identified and thus the care they need is not being provided. In the latter case, cost-effectiveness is minimal because many individuals are given treatment that they may not need. This is not necessarily harmful, since the treatment typically involves more prenatal care. However, for maximum cost-effectiveness and outcome effectiveness, it is critical that perinatal risk scores be set at a level that will ensure accurate classification of individuals being assessed.

Hobel (1980) discussed the importance of specificity and sensitivity in an article on changes in rates of high-risk pregnancy. He noted that the classification system he has used, in which women with scores of 10 or higher are classified as "high risk," has, in recent years, been identifying more women in that category. Between 1972 and 1978, the percent of high-risk pregnancies identified under Hobel's system rose from 32% to 64%. The sensitivity rate also increase, from 50% to 83%, but specificity decreased, from 70% to 20%. Thus, although more abnormal cases were identified as being "at risk," fewer of the normal cases were identified as being "not at risk." Hobel noted that the sensitivity rate had become so high that it would be difficult to provide the highest quality prenatal care to so many women. In an effort to reduce the sensitivity rate and to increase the specificity rate, Hobel proposed changing the high-risk cutoff score used with his scale from 10 to 25. He also examined the individual conditions on the scale, to determine if there had been changes over the 6-year time span in predictive validity. He found that some conditions that were predictive of negative outcomes in 1972 (e.g., severe pre-eclampsia, heavy meconium, abnormal presentation) were no longer preditive in 1978 and that some new conditions were identified as predictive in 1978 (e.g., history of previous stillbirth, shoulder dystocia). He attributed these shifts to changes both in the obstetric population and in clinical practices and available interventions.

Wilson and Shifrin (1980) have pointed out that it may be difficult to set a safe specificity level because of the uncertainty of risks that might arise in seemingly normal, "low-risk" pregnancies and labors. These authors worry that orienting perinatal risk scores toward greater sensitivity will be at the expense of missing the potential risks inherent in pregnancies that are other than "high risk." This concern has also been expressed by other researchers (Lesinski, 1975, Sylvain, 1984). Clearly, rigid adherence to perinatal risk categories based on scores alone is not likely to produce satisfactory results. In assigning patients to perinatal risk categories, physicians must also use clinical judgment and must be sure that the categories are valid for use with the obstetric population to which it is being applied. Such a system is most likely to produce successful results—that is, accurate identification of perinatal risk.

SUMMARY

Perinatal risk screening scales are a means by which to assess medical histories and the medical conditions arising in patients and research subjects during the antepartum, intrapartum, and postpartum periods. Ideally, perinatal risk scales should permit information from medical records to be quantified easily and accurately, so that the resultant scores can be used to predict the risk of a poor outcome during the perinatal period and of abnormal development during infancy and childhood. A number of perinatal risk scales have been developed that are designed to screen for complications during the antepartum, intrapartum, and postpartum periods. These scales have been found to differ on a number of dimensions, including the defining characteristics by which complications are assessed, the scores that are assigned to specific risk conditions, and the use of the scores in assigning individuals to risk categories. In addition, questions have been raised concerning (1) the validity of the scales in screening subjects in obstetric and pediatric populations other than those for which the scales were developed and (2) the relative performance across scales in accurately predicting perinatal outcomes. These issues regarding the validity and predictive accuracy of the scales are addressed in the chapters that follow.

CHAPTER

2

Perinatal Risk Screening Scales

In the previous chapter, several different types of scales for screening perinatal risk were described and the general characteristics of each type were discussed. In this chapter, the focus narrows to six perinatal risk scales that have been used in research and clinical studies and that are prominent in the literature. The discussion of these scales will focus on the items they contain, the weighting systems used, the risk points used in assigning risk categories, how the scales were developed, their validity and reliability (if known), how the scales have been utilized in research and clinical studies, and what types of outcome measures have been used with them. The six scales chosen for this discussion were developed by Brazie *et al.* (cited in Lubchenco, 1976), Hobel *et al.* (1973), Littman and Parmelee (1978), Aubry and colleagues (Nesbitt & Aubry, 1969; Aubry & Pennington, 1973), Prechtl (1967), and Zax *et al.* (1977).

The six scales share a number of similar characteristics. First, they are uncomplicated, objective scoring systems that can be readily scored by using the defining characteristics contained on the scale or provided separately by the scale developers or by using information available in the research literature. Second, each scale contains items that can be scored on the basis of information drawn from medical records. Medical records are an important source of perinatal information, particularly in retrospective studies, in which the perinatal risk scales are scored exclusively on the basis of information taken from medical records during the postpartum period. Since medical records are often heavily utilized in prospective studies as well, these scales seem to adapt well to various research designs.

Third, these scales are composed of items pertaining to antepartum, intrapartum, and postpartum phenomena. The items contained on the scales have a known or a commonly assumed relationship to perinatal complications. Thus there are few items whose value in predicting perinatal risk is controversial. Fourth, these scales all contain item weightings based on the developers' understanding of the relative significance of each item or on risk norms derived from studies of large samples. Fifth, each scale is composed of items that have clear defining characteristics, so that risk scores can be assigned to each item and converted into total scale scores, subscale score, or both.

In contrast to these similarities, the scales vary in several important ways. First, they differ in the number of antepartum, intrapartum, and postpartum items they contain and in the types of complications represented by the items. The number of items on the scales ranges from as few as 25 to as many as 126. These items represent perinatal conditions that are generally contained on perinatal risk scales, but some of the conditions are uniquely represented on only some scales. Second, there are differences across scales in the defining characteristics used with each item to assign risk. Third, there are differences across scales in the scores assigned to specific conditions. Finally, these scales have been developed for use in different types of situations, some for use in clinical settings, and others for use in research studies of behavioral assessment and child development. The performance of these scales in situations other than those for which they were developed is often unknown. Because such differences exist among the scales, there is reason to expect that there will be differences in their predictive validity. Such differences in predictive validity could provide a basis for selecting one scale over another for a particular reseach or clinical purpose.

In the discussion that follows, each of the six perinatal risk scales is described in detail and is shown in an accompanying table. Issues related to the validity of each scale are explored in relation to the types of research and clinical settings in which each scale has been applied.

UNIVERSITY OF COLORADO NEONATAL MORBIDITY RISK SCALE

The University of Colorado Neonatal Morbidity Risk Scale (UCNM), developed by Brazie *et al.* (cited in Lubchenco, 1976) and shown in Table 2-1, has 25 items, 15 pertaining to the antepartum period, 7 to the intrapartum period, and 3 to the neonate. The score assigned to each item is based on the empirically determined probability of the complication represented by the item resulting in infant morbidity. The risk probabilities are based on data obtained from a University of Colorado Medical Center study of 3,487 women and their infants. These probabilities range from –8.5 to 40.7 points and vary on the basis of the use of antenatal information only or the use of antepartum, intrapartum, and newborn information. Scores are summed to obtain a total morbidity risk score. No risk category scores are reported. Reliability estimates have not been reported by the scale developers.

Reports on the validity of the UCNM have pertained more to the validity of the specific items on the scale than to the validity of the total score. No reports were found in the literature of the use of this whole scale in any research or clinical studies other than those by Molfese and colleagues (Molfese & Thomson, 1985; Molfese *et al.,* 1985; Molfese, Thomson, Beadnell, Bricker, & Manion, 1987). The absence of other reports is surprising, since this is the only published scale that uses exact risk probabilities for scale weights, which would seem to make it a likely scale to use in comparisons with other scales that use more arbitrarily assigned weights.

One aspect of the Brazie *et al.* scale that has been validated is the birthweight–gestational age morbidity score and mortality score. In an earlier article, Lubchenco, Searls, and Brazie (1972) reported on the value of using birthweight and gestational age in predicting both morbidity and mortality rates. Over a 10-year period, 14,436 births and 341 neonatal deaths were studied. Both morbidity and mortality rates were noted to vary with birthweight and gestational age. Lower morbidity and mortality rates were noted for heavier infants at all gestational

TABLE 2-1. Brazie, Searls, and Lubchenco's University of Colorado Neonatal Morbidity Risk Scale

Obstetric history	Risk based on antenatal information only (% risk)	Risk based on antenatal and intrapartum information and on immediate condition of newborn (% risk)
Previous neonatal death	8.1	
Previous low birthweight infant	5.1	
Mother's age <17 yr	6.0	
Incompetent cervix	32.5	
Placenta previa, abruptio placentae, antepartum hemorrhage	31.0	
Attempted abortion, suicide, drug intoxication	13.8	
Prolapsed cord	17.1	
Breech position	13.5	
Other labor complications[a]	27.2	23.8
Abnormal presentation at delivery	24.6	10.7
Maternal diabetes	40.7	33.3
Rh and other isoimmunization	39.4	34.5
Abdominal and/or major surgery, accident, antepartum	30.5	14.0
Premature rupture of membranes	27.6	12.3
Toxemia	22.4	14.0
Amniocentesis	7.8	6.6
Multiple gestation	7.2	−8.5
Prenatal care: none	9.4	4.2
1 to 3 visits	7.6	3.8
4 to 7 visits	4.4	3.0
8+ visits	1.3	2.2
Fetal distress	11.5	5.2
Cesarean section	10.5	5.5
Other delivery complications		10.4
Mother's age >30 yr		2.7
Male infant		1.8
Active resuscitation, delivery room		8.3
Birthweight–gestational age morbidity score = (from Figure 2-2)		☐
Total	☐	Total ☐

Note. To obtain antenatal risk score, circle the items that apply and add circled numbers. To obtain risk after birth, circle numbers of items that apply and add the birthweight–gestational age score from Figure 2-2. From *The High Risk Infant* by L. O. Lubchenco, 1976. Philadelphia: W. B. Saunders, p. 120. Copyright 1976 by W. B. Saunders Co. Reprinted by permission.

[a]Induction, Pitocin stimulation, uterine inertia, contracted pelvis, shock.

ages and for infants with longer gestational ages at all birthweights over 500 grams. The mortality rates are reflected in the scores shown in Figures 2-1 and 2-2. The use of both birthweight and gestational age is noted by the authors to be one means of screening large populations of infants that does not require inclusion of other perinatal risk factors. Table 2-2 can be used as a means of predicting level of morbidity and mortality risk involved.

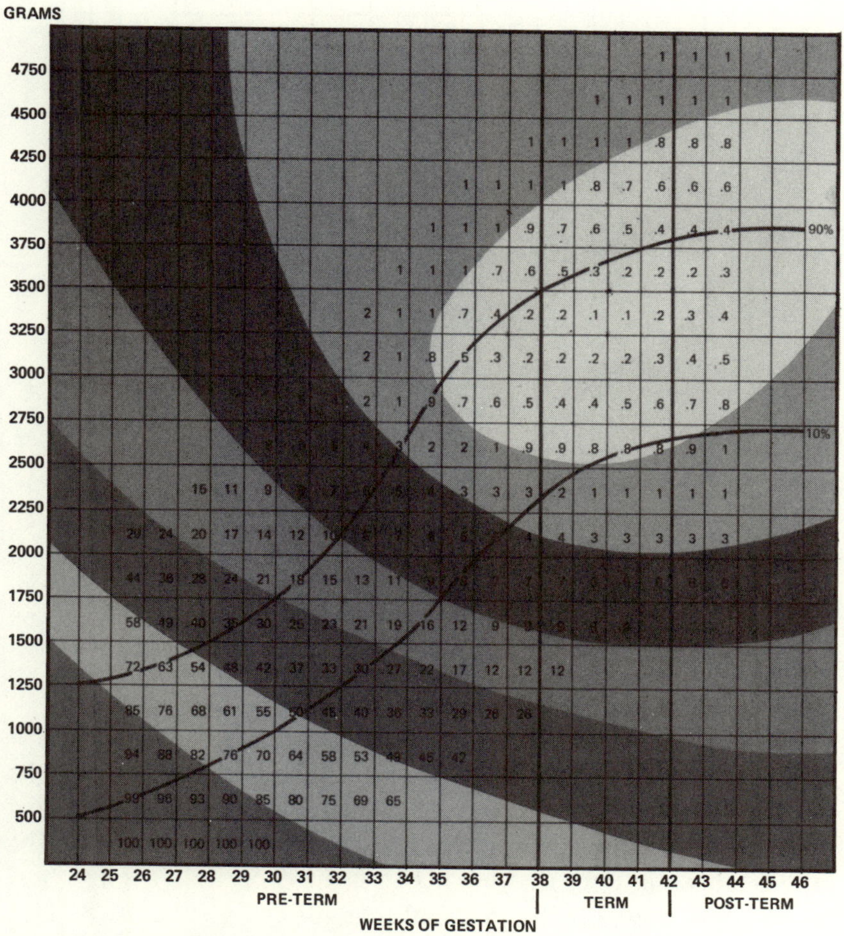

FIGURE 2-1. Neonatal birthweight–gestational age mortality risk scores. From *The High Risk Infant* by L. O. Lubchenco, 1976. Philadelphia: W. B. Saunders, p. 105. Copyright 1976 by W. B. Saunders Co. Reprinted by permission.

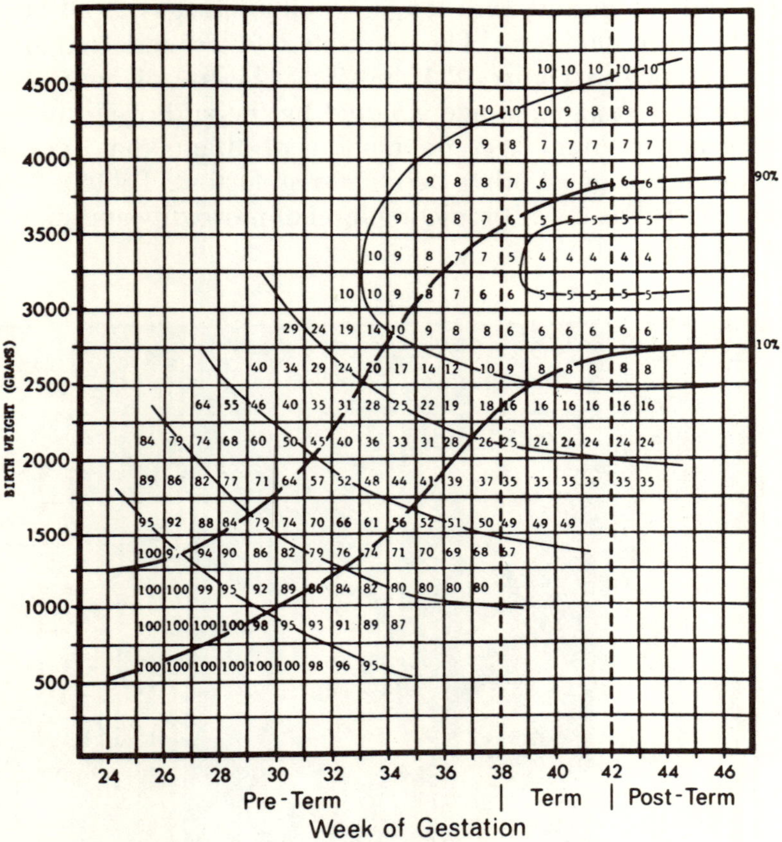

FIGURE 2-2. Neonatal morbidity risk by birthweight–gestational age. From *The High Risk Infant* by L. O. Lubchenco, 1976. Philadelphia: W. B. Saunders, p. 113. Copyright 1976 by W. B. Saunders Co. Reprinted by permission.

The two-factor (birthweight and gestational age) risk score was modified for inclusion in the UCNM. The birthweight morbidity risk score (shown in Table 2-2) is calculated by multiplying the neonatal morbidity risk score (based on birthweight and gestational age, as shown in Figure 2-2) by .76 and then adding risk points if the 5-minute Apgar score is below 8. The score thus obtained is part of the total UCNM, but the authors also seem to suggest that this score alone might be useful for predicting infant morbidity. The birthweight–gestational age

TABLE 2-2. Brazie, Searls, and Lubchencho's Postpartum Morbidity and Mortality Risk Scores

Morbidity risk		
Birthweight–gestational age morbidity risk[a] × .76	=	☐
Apgar score (5 min)		
8–10	=	0
5–7	=	16.5
0–4	=	33.0
Total % chance of becoming ill	=	☐

Mortality risk		
Birthweight–gestational age mortality risk[b] × .75	=	☐
Apgar score (5 min)		
8–10	=	0
5–7	=	11.0
0–4	=	22.0
Total % chance of dying	=	☐

Note. From *The High Risk Infant* by L. O. Lubchenco, 1976. Philadelphia: W. B. Saunders, p. 121. Copyright 1976 by W. B. Saunders Co. Reprinted by permission.

[a]Birthweight–gestational age morbidity risk obtained from Figure 2-2.

[b]Birthweight–gestational age mortality risk obtained from Figure 2-1.

mortality risk score (shown in Table 2-2) also might be useful alone. The validity of this portion of the scale has not been reported.

HIGH-RISK PREGNANCY SCREENING SYSTEM

The High-Risk Pregnancy Screening System (HRPSS), developed by Hobel *et al.* (1973), contains items that were obtained from other perinatal risk scales or that were derived from the authors' clinical experiences. The 126 items are grouped into three categories: prenatal (51 items), intrapartum (40 items), and neonatal (35 items). Each item is assigned a score of 1, 5, or 10, based on its assumed value in predicting morbidity and mortality. Item scores are summed in order to obtain total and subscale scores. Scores less than 10 indicate "low risk," and scores of 10 or greater, "high risk." The original Hobel *et al.* scale—the HRPSS (shown in Table 2-3)—was later reconfigured into the Problem-Oriented Perinatal Risk Assessment System (POPRAS) (one section of which is shown in Table 2-4), which is widely used as a perinatal screening device in medical centers. Compared to the HRPSS, the POPRAS contains some different items as well as an extensive list of mater-

TABLE 2-3. Hobel, Hyvarinen, Okada, and Oh's (1973) High-Risk Pregnancy Screening System

		Score
	Prenatal factors	
I.	Cardiovascular and renal	
	1. Moderate to severe toxemia	10
	2. Chronic hypertension	10
	3. Moderate to severe renal disease	10
	4. Severe heart disease, Class II–IV	10
	5. History of eclampsia	5
	6. History of pyelitis	5
	7. Class I heart disease	5
	8. Mild toxemia	5
	9. Acute pyelonephritis	5
	10. History of cystitis	1
	11. Acute cystitis	1
	12. History of toxemia	1
II.	Metabolic	
	1. Diabetes ≥ Class A-II	10
	2. Previous endocrine ablation	10
	3. Thyroid disease	5
	4. Prediabetes (A-I)	5
	5. Family history of diabetes	1
III.	Previous histories	
	1. Previous fetal exchange transfusion for Rh	10
	2. Previous stillbirth	10
	3. Post-term >42 wk	10
	4. Previous premature infant	10
	5. Previous neonatal death	10
	6. Previous cesarean section	5
	7. Habitual abortion	5
	8. Infant > 10 lb	5
	9. Multiparity > 5	5
	10. Epilepsy	5
	11. Fetal anomalies	1

(*continued*)

TABLE 2-3. *(Continued)*

		Score
IV.	Anatomic abnormalities	
	1. Uterine malformation	10
	2. Incompetent cervix	10
	3. Abnormal fetal position	10
	4. Polyhydramnios	10
	5. Small pelvis	5
V.	Miscellaneous	
	1. Abnormal cervical cytology	10
	2. Multiple pregnancy	10
	3. Sickle cell disease	10
	4. Age $\geq$ 35 or $\leq$ 15 yr	5
	5. Viral disease	5
	6. Rh sensitization only	5
	7. Positive serology	5
	8. Severe anemia (< 9 gm Hb)	5
	9. Excessive use of drugs	5
	10. History of TB or PPD $\geq$ 10mm	5
	11. Weight < 100 or > 200 lb	5
	12. Pulmonary disease	5
	13. Flu syndrome (severe)	5
	14. Vaginal spotting	5
	15. Mild anemia (9–10.9 gm Hb)	1
	16. Smoking $\geq$ 1 pack per day	1
	17. Alcohol (moderate)	1
	18. Emotional problem	1

	Intrapartum factors	
I.	Maternal factors	
	1. Moderate–severe toxemia	10
	2. Hydramnios or oligohydramnios	10
	3. Amnionitis	10
	4. Uterine rupture	10
	5. Mild toxemia	5
	6. Premature rupture of membrane > 12 hr	5
	7. Primary dysfunctional labor	5
	8. Secondary arrest of dilation	5
	9. Demerol > 300 mg	5
	10. $MgSO_4$ > 25 gm	5
	11. Labor > 20 hr	5
	12. Second stage > 2½ hr	5
	13. Clinical small pelvis	5
	14. Medical induction	5
	15. Precipitous labor < 3 hr	5
	16. Primary cesarean section	5

(continued)

TABLE 2-3. *(Continued)*

		Score
	17. Repeat cesarean section	5
	18. Elective induction	1
	19. Prolonged latent phase	1
	20. Uterine tetany	1
	21. Pitocin augmentation	1
II.	Placental factors	
	1. Placenta previa	10
	2. Abruptio placentae	10
	3. Post-term > 42 wk	10
	4. Meconium-stained amniotic fluid (dark)	10
	5. Meconium-stained amniotic fluid (light)	5
	6. Marginal separation	1
III.	Fetal factors	
	1. Abnormal presentation	10
	2. Multiple pregnancy	10
	3. Fetal bradycardia > 30 min	10
	4. Breech delivery—total extraction	10
	5. Prolapsed cord	10
	6. Fetal weight < 2,500 gm	10
	7. Fetal acidosis—pH ≤ 7.25 (Stage I)	10
	8. Fetal tachycardia > 30 min	10
	9. Operative forceps or vacuum extraction	5
	10. Breech delivery—spontaneous or assisted	5
	11. General anesthesia	5
	12. Outlet forceps	1
	13. Shoulder dystocia	1

	Neonatal factors	
I.	General	
	1. Prematurity < 2,000 gm	10
	2. Apgar at 5 min < 5	10
	3. Resuscitation at birth	10
	4. Fetal anomalies	10
	5. Dysmaturity	5
	6. Prematurity < 2,000–2,500 gm	5
	7. Apgar at 1 min < 5	5
	8. Feeding problem	1
	9. Multiple birth	1
II.	Respiratory	
	1. Respiratory distress syndrome	10
	2. Meconium aspiration syndrome	10
	3. Congenital pneumonia	10
	4. Anomalies of respiratory system	10

(*continued*)

TABLE 2-3. *(Continued)*

		Score
	5. Apnea	10
	6. Other respiratory distress	10
	7. Transient tachypnea	5
III.	Metabolic disorders	
	1. Hypoglycemia	10
	2. Hypocalcemia	10
	3. Hypomagnesemia or hypermagnesemia	5
	4. Hypoparathyroidism	5
	5. Failure to gain weight	1
	6. Jitteriness or hyperactivity with specific causes	1
IV.	Cardiac	
	1. Major cardiac anomalies requiring immediate catheterization	10
	2. CHF	10
	3. Persistent cyanosis	5
	4. Cardiac anomalies not requiring immediate catheterization	5
	5. Murmur	5
V.	Hematologic problems	
	1. Hyperbilirubinemia	10
	2. Hemorrhagic diathesis	10
	3. Chromosomal anomalies	10
	4. Sepsis	10
	5. Anemia	5
VI.	Central nervous system	
	1. CNS depression > 24 hr	10
	2. Seizures	10
	3. CNS depression < 24 hr	5

Note. PPD = purified protein derivative of tuberculin; $MgSO_4$ = magnesium sulfate; CHF = congestive heart failure; CNS = central nervous system. From "Prenatal and Intrapartum High-Risk Screening: I. Prediction of the High-Risk Neonate" by C. J. Hobel, M. A. Hyvarinen, D. M. Okada, and W. Oh, 1973. *American Journal of Obstetrics and Gynecology, 117,* pp. 2–4. Copyright 1973 by C. V. Mosby Co. Reprinted by permission.

nal postpartum items. The maternal postpartum items are unweighted, however, which does not permit a risk score to be derived from them. Reliability estimates for both the HRPSS and the POPRAS have not been reported.

Hobel *et al.* (1973) evaluated the validity of the antepartum and intrapartum subscales of the HRPSS. The outcome measures were the neonatal scores from the scale, the length of the infant's hospital stay, 1- and 5-minute Apgar scores, and infant

TABLE 2-4. "Prenatal History" Section of Hobel, Hyvarinen, Okada, and Oh's Problem-Oriented Perinatal Risk Assessment System

Patient Address			
City	State	Zip	Birth Date
Home Phone	Preferred Language	Marital Status M W D SEP S	
Contact Phone	Race-Ethnicity W B H I A O	Spouse's Name	
Referred By	Hospital of Delivery		

INTAKE DATE & INITIALS:

PAST PREGNANCIES

OB INDEX

Age	Term	Premi	Ab-Ectop	Living

BIRTH CONTROL PILLS IN PAST YEAR ☐ Yes ☐ No

MENSES Onset / Int / Dur

CYCLES ☐ Regular ☐ Irregular

LMP: ☐ Normal ☐ Abnormal PMP:

EDC:

POSITIVE PREGNANCY TEST Date:

Pregnancy No.	Termination Date Mo.	Termination Date Yr.	Early Loss <20 wks Spon	Early Loss <20 wks Ectop	Early Loss <20 wks Induced*	GA wks	≥20 wks Live or Stillborn Birth Wt	Sex	Living Y/N**	Vaginal Spon Vtx	Vaginal Br	Vaginal Forceps	C-Section CPD	C-Section Fetal Distress	C-Section Abn Pres	C-Section Repeat	C-Section Other/Unk	Associated Problems
1																		
2																		
3																		
4																		
5																		
6																		
7																		
8																		

*D&C S(Suction) Sa(Saline) P(Prostaglandin) H(Hysterotomy) O(Other) U(Unknown) **S(Stillbirth) N(Neonatal) I(Infant) C(Childhood)

HISTORICAL PROBLEMS

Prob. No.	±	Risk Value		
1		5		☐ AGE <17 ☐ AGE ≥35
2		5		MULTIPARITY (5 or more ≥20 weeks)
3		5		INDUCED ABORTION
4		10		HABITUAL ABORTION (3 or more)
5		10	PREVIOUS INFANTS	PREMATURE (<37 weeks) ☐ LGA
6		10		SGA (Small for Gestational Age)
7		5		BIRTH WEIGHT >4000 gms or 9 lbs
8		10		PERINATAL DEATH ☐ Stillborn ☐ Neonatal
9		5		POST NEONATAL PROBLEM ☐ Sudden Infant Death ☐ Neurologic Handicap ☐ Mental Retardation
10		10		NEONATAL JAUNDICE ☐ Rh ☐ ABO ☐ Physiologic ☐ Unknown ☐ Other:
11		5		GENETIC DISEASE ☐ Chromosomal ☐ CNS ☐ Inborn Errors of Metabolism ☐ Other: ☐ Structural Congenital Anomalies:
12		5	GYN	HISTORY OF INFERTILITY ☐ Primary ☐ Secondary ☐ Treated ☐ Untreated
13		10		UTERINE-CERVICAL ABNORMALITY ☐ Uterine Anomaly ☐ Corrected ☐ Incomp Cx ☐ Cerclage, Removed ☐ Yes ☐ No
14		5		PREVIOUS UTERINE SURGERY C-Section: ☐ Classical ☐ Low Trans ☐ Low Vert ☐ Unknown ☐ Hysterotomy ☐ Myomectomy
15		5	PREG. COMPLICATIONS	HEMORRHAGE ☐ Previa ☐ Abruptio ☐ Other 3rd Trimester ☐ Post Partum ☐ Transfusion
16		5		PREGNANCY-INDUCED HYPERTENSION ☐ Required Hosp ☐ Required Early Delivery ☐ Developed Eclampsia
17		10	MEDICAL-SURGICAL	CHRONIC HYPERTENSION (BP ≥140/90 non-pregnant) ☐ On Drug Therapy:
18		10		HEART DISEASE ☐ Rheumatic ☐ Congenital ☐ Arteriosclerotic ☐ Other ☐ Surgical Correction ☐ Hx of CHF or Arrhythmia ☐ No limitation of physical activity ☐ Slight limitation ☐ Marked limitation ☐ Unable to carry on any physical activ. w/out discomfort
19		5		PULMONARY DISEASE ☐ Asthma ☐ Chronic Bronchitis ☐ Tuberculosis ☐ Other
20		5		GENITOURINARY INFECTIONS ☐ Asymptomatic Bacteruria ☐ Cystitis ☐ Pyelonephritis ☐ Gonorrhea ☐ Syphilis ☐ Genital Herpes
21		10		RENAL DISEASE ☐ Glomerulo ☐ Chronic Pyelo ☐ Diabetic ☐ Collagen-vas ☐ Calculi ☐ Other:
22		10		DIABETES ☐ A ☐ B ☐ C ☐ D ☐ F-R ☐ Insulin, Pre-preg Dosage:
23		10		THYROID DISEASE ☐ Hypo ☐ Thyroiditis ☐ Hyper: treated with ☐ Drugs ☐ Surgery ☐ I-131
24		10		OTHER MEDICAL ☐ Phlebitis ☐ Embolus ☐ Collagen-vas ☐ On Drug Therapy: ☐ Hematologic:
25		10		EPILEPSY ☐ On Therapy: ☐ Phenobarb ☐ Dilantin ☐ Mysoline ☐ Other:
26		5		PSYCHIATRIC ☐ Hospitalized ☐ On Drug Therapy:
27		5		PREVIOUS OPERATIONS ☐ Diag D&C ☐ Laparoscopy ☐ Appendectomy ☐ Cholecystectomy ☐ Other:
28		10	HABITS	EXCESSIVE USE ☐ Alcohol ☐ Tobacco ☐ Marijuana ☐ Narcotics:
29		5	FAMILY HISTORY	MATERNAL ONLY ☐ Hypertension ☐ Multiple Births ☐ Diabetes ☐ Hemoglobinopathy ☐ DES ☐ Other:
30		5		MAT. OR PATERNAL ☐ Mental Retardation ☐ Congen Anom ☐ Congen Hearing Loss ☐ Allergies ☐ Other:

HEALTH STATUS INDICATORS

YEARS OF EDUCATION Mother______ Father______

DIET (Ex, G, P, Undet) Calories______ Protein______ Iron______

INSURANCE ☐ Public ☐ Private ☐ None

Carrier______ #______ #______

Carrier______ #______ #______

ALLERGIES

COMMENTS

SPECIAL COMMENTS FOR DATA ENTRY

1 PRENATAL HISTORY

Note. Adapted from "Prenatal and Intrapartum High-Risk Screening: I. Prediction of the High-Risk Neonate" by C. J. Hobel, M. A. Hyvarinen, D. M. Okada, and W. Oh, 1973. *American Journal of Obstetrics and Gynecology, 117*, pp. 1–9. Copyright 1973 by C. V. Mosby Co. Adapted by permission.

mortality. A prospective sample of 725 women was used in the study. Hobel *et al.* noted that most subjects had had at least one risk condition. Women with high antepartum and high intrapartum (HIGH/HIGH) scores on the HRPSS were found to have a neonatal morbidity rate of 35% and a perinatal mortality rate of 14.5%. Women with low antepartum and low intrapartum (LOW/LOW) scores had a neonatal morbidity rate of 6.5% and a perinatal mortality rate of .0004%. Women with high antepartum and low intrapartum (HIGH/LOW) scores had morbidity and mortality rates of 11.8% and .022%, respectively. Women with low antepartum and high intrapartum (LOW/HIGH) scores had morbidity and mortality rates of 24.3% and .035%, respectively. In general, sensitivity was greatest for women with high intrapartum risk scores. Intrapartum scores were also found to be more accurate than antepartum scores in predicting the length of the infants' hospital stay.

Sokol *et al.* (1977) provided validity data on the HRPSS in a study that screened 1,275 consecutive maternity patients for perinatal risk. In using the Hobel *et al.* cutoff scores to divide the patients into "low-risk" and "high-risk" categories, these researchers classified 30.5% of the patients as having low antepartum and low intrapartum (LOW/LOW) risk, 23% as having high antepartum and low intrapartum (HIGH/LOW) risk, 20.5% as having low antepartum and high intrapartum (LOW/HIGH) risk, and 26% as having high antepartum and high intrapartum (HIGH/HIGH) risk. Compared with the Hobel *et al.* study, Sokol *et al.* found more LOW/LOW and HIGH/LOW women and fewer HIGH/HIGH women in their sample. Sokol *et al.* also found that scores on the antepartum and intrapartum subscales were significantly correlated with 1- and 5-minute Apgar scores and with perinatal infant death. Patients with low antepartum and intrapartum scores had significantly higher 1- and 5-minute Apgar scores than did patients with high scores during the antepartum period, the intrapartum period, or both periods. All perinatal deaths occurred in infants of patients with high scores on at least one subscale, with 81.6% of the deaths occurring in infants of patients who had high antepartum and intrapartum subscale scores. A result similar to the finding of the Hobel *et al.* study was that sensitivity was greatest for patients with high intrapartum risk scores.

Baruffi *et al.* (1984) examined the validity of the "high-risk" definition used by Hobel *et al.* According to Hobel *et al.*, women receiving a score of 10 points or more on the scale were classified as "high risk." In the Baruffi *et al.* study, samples of women from two different hospitals were obtained. One sample was composed of 796 women, and the other, of 804 women. Scores on the HRPSS neonatal subscale were used as the dependent variables. Three different definitions of "high risk" were used: scores over 10, scores over 15, and scores over 20. The two samples, though similar in social and demographic characteristics, were found to differ in antepartum and intrapartum risks, so that none of the three definitions used to classify women as "high risk" was useful for predicting neonatal morbidity in both populations. The authors noted that modifications in risk score categories might be necessary when the scale is used with different obstetric populations.

Use of the HRPSS in Various Studies

Other researchers have incorporated the HRPSS into various types of research investigations. Johnson, Krejci, Hack, and Fanaroff (1984) used the HRPSS in a study of enamel defects in the incisors of very low birthweight infants. No significant correlations were found between enamel defects and HRPSS scores, gestational age, birthweight, or caloric intake by the mother. Cox, Hack, and Metz (1984) studied auditory brain-stem responses in very low birthweight infants. Abnormalities in brain-stem responses were significantly associated with HRPSS scores. Further, it was found that the neonatal scores from the scale could be used to discriminate accurately between infants with and infants without abnormalities in brain-stem responses. Interestingly, scale scores were more predictive of abnormalities in brain-stem responses than were individual risk conditions. Gross *et al.* (1980) examined pregnancy risk and neonatal outcome in 270 obese women. Few differences in labor complications or neonatal outcome measures were noted between the women who were obese and those who were not. However, the obese group did have more antepartum risks, along with fewer low birthweight and more meconium-stained infants. Eskes, Timmer, Kollee, and Jongsma (1985) studied the effect of perinatal variables on second-born versus firstborn members of twin pairs. The HRPSS was used to quantify antepartum complications. Although female sex, maternal menstrual onset at a young age, low birthweight, and instrument delivery were found to be predictors of lower Apgar scores and of acidemia in the umbilical artery, parity and antepartum risk scores were not significantly related to these outcome measures.

In contrast to its use as a predictor variable in the preceding studies, the HRPSS has been used as a means of characterizing subjects in studies of infant development. Luz (1985) used the scale in a study of auditory evoked responses in 233 human fetuses during the intrapartum period. The Hobel *et al.* criteria were used to divide the fetuses into "risk" and "no-risk" categories. Sounds of 1,500 hertz were used to evoke motoric and heart-rate responses in the fetuses. Although no significant differences were noted in motor behaviors between the "risk" and "no-risk" fetus groups, there were significant differences between the groups in duration of heart-rate acceleration, initial increase in heart rate, maximum increase in heart rate, and mean heart rate. Interestingly, only 19 of the 233 fetuses had no risk factors. Luz suggested that greater sensitivity might be achieved by the use of more than two categories of risk.

Friedman (1982) used the HRPSS with (1) a group of 45 preterm infants who were classified by scores on the scale as being at "low medical risk" and (2) a group of 23 healthy, full-term neonates. The study focused on the role played by the behavioral style of infants in their interactions with caregivers. The researchers found that preterm infants were more irritable, needed more soothing intervention, and changed states more often than full-term neonates. These demanding characteristics tended to make caregiving more difficult. In a separate study, Friedman, Jacobs, and Werthmann (1982) examined the aversiveness of preterm and full-term infants' cries to maternal perception and responsiveness. Scores on the HRPSS were again used to identify those infants who were at "low medical risk." The results were interpreted as showing that preterm infants' cries were not perceived as more negative than those of full-term infants.

The HRPSS has also been studied for its value as an antenatal screening system when incorporated into hospital settings. Sokol *et al.* (1980) used the scale to screen patients participating in a special maternity and infant care prenatal program. Those women who participated in the program had lower perinatal mortality rates than nonparticipants. Lilford and Chard (1982) reported on an effort that utilized a computer-based model to maximize the effectiveness of the HRPSS as a screening device in antepartum care. The researchers examined all medical records entered into the new system. Of the perinatal deaths, 80% occurred in the group scoring as "high risk" on the HRPSS. Unter (1982) used scores from the scale as a method of predicting perinatal risks and complications in a sample of infants who were involved in a program to transport those considered "high risk" to a regional facility for intensive care. Bukovsky *et al.* (1985) used the HRPSS as a means of identifying high-risk pregnancies in an effort to determine what effect a physicians' strike might have on the incidence of such pregnancies. The incidence of these pregnancies before, during, and after the strike was found to be unchanged. Rishpon, Epstein, and Egoz (1985) utilized scores from the scale to screen for prenatal risk in a study of the effects of a prenatal care program. Infants who died within 1 year of birth were found to have had higher antepartum risk scores on the scale compared to infants who did not die.

Two studies have provided validity data on the POPRAS. First, Hobel (1980) reported on a group of subjects whose antepartum and intrapartum risks were assessed at 2-year intervals between 1972 and 1978 using POPRAS criteria, with scores less than 10 indicating "low risk" and those greater than 10, "high risk." Over the time period studied, a steady decrease was noted in the number of subjects classified as "low risk" in both the antepartum and the intrapartum periods (LOW/LOW) and in those classified as "low risk" in the antepartum period and as "high risk" in the intrapartum period (LOW/HIGH). Increases were noted in the number of subjects classified as "high risk" in the antepartum period and as "low risk" in both the intrapartum period (HIGH/LOW) and in those classified as "high risk" in both periods (HIGH/HIGH). Hobel also noted that sensitivity increased over time from 50% to 83% but that specificity decreased from 70% to 20%. He offered two suggestions that were aimed at increasing the specificity rate and decreasing the sensitivity rate to more manageable levels. Based on changes noted over the study period (1972 to 1978) in the relationship between percent of "high-risk" infants and antepartum risk scores, Hobel recommended that the antepartum "high-risk" cutoff score on the POPRAS be raised from greater than 10 to greater than 25. By using "greater than 25" as a cutoff score, the number of high-risk patients identified would be approximately equal to the number identified as such in 1972 using a cutoff score of "greater than 10." Hobel also recommended that because of changes in the predictive validity of specific perinatal risk scale items over time, changes be made periodically in these items used to screen patients.

The second study providing validity data on the POPRAS was that conducted by Campbell and Wilhelm (1985), who examined the development of high-risk infants. A sample of 15 infants was studied to determine if POPRAS scores could be used as predictors of infants who would be at risk for developmental abnormalities, to determine how early in development such abnormalities could be identified, and to document development during the first year of life. The infants studied had POPRAS scores of over 50 points and at least four of the following complications: 5-minute Apgar scores of 5 or under, resuscitation at birth, asphyxia, repeated apnea, persistent cyanosis, hyperbilirubinemia requiring an exchange transfusion, systemic viral or bacterial infection, central nervous system depression longer than 24 hours, seizures, jitteriness, central nervous system hemorrhage or infarction, and skull fracture. Measures were obtained on the Brazelton Neonatal Behavioral Assessment Scale, the Bayley Scales of Infant Development, the Denver Developmental Screening Test, the Stanford–Binet, and the Home Observation for Measurement of Environment (HOME) Scale (Caldwell & Bradley, 1978), and on a variety of motor assessment scales. The result of the study was that the POPRAS scores permitted the correct identification of 80% of the infants who had developmental problems. Thus the POPRAS seemed to have a good sensitivity rate. Interestingly, motor performance at age 3 months was the best single early predictor of neurological outcome at 3 years of age. This measure produced a correct identification rate of 89%.

The neonatal subscale from the HRPSS has been used in a variety of other studies. For example, Strobino and Baruffi (1984) evaluated its use as a measure of infant morbidity by examining issues of internal consistency, criterion validity, and weightings of risk items. Internal consistency was examined by determining both the percent distribution of the number of items (conditions) for infants with each item (condition) and the proportion of infants with a given item (condition) for infants with one or more conditions. If the scores were internally consistent, infants with one condition would also have other conditions. Criterion validity of the scores was determined by using the length of hospital stay as a measure of outcome status. Weightings of risk items were examined by determining whether the conditions (risk items) with the heavier weightings were more likely to co-occur with other conditions than were conditions with lesser weightings. Data from a sample of 1,600 infants were used. The authors reported that the neonatal risk score was internally consistent, with all items occurring with some frequency and in conjunction with at least one other item. Thus the conditions, or complications, represented by the items seem to give rise to other complications. The items were also generally found to distinguish between infants with high scores and those with low scores. The neonatal scores were highly correlated with length of hospital stay (r = .67). Thus the scores generated by the HRPSS neonatal subscale were interpreted to be valid predictors of these indicators of infant morbidity.

The HRPSS neonatal subscale was used by Cox, Hack, and Metz (1981) to characterize a sample of 40 high-risk preterm infants. These infants, all of whom had low neonatal risk scores, were in a study to evaluate the use of brain-stem evoked response audiometry. Brain-stem evoked response audiometry was found to be a reliable measure of auditory functioning in these infants.

OBSTETRICAL COMPLICATIONS SCALE

The Obstetrical Complications Scale (OCS) (Littman & Parmelee, 1978) is based on Prechtl's (1967) optimal scoring system and contains all but one of the items on the Prechtl Scale of Optimal Obstetric Conditions, which is described later in this chapter. The OCS (shown in Table 2-5) contains 41 items, 20 pertaining to the antepartum period, 15 to the intrapartum period, and 6 to the infant. Items are scored as "optimal = 1" or "nonoptimal = 0," and scores are summed to obtain a total

TABLE 2-5. Littman and Parmelee's (1978) Obstetrical Complications Scale

Infant's name ________________________________

Hospital number ________________________________

Birth date ____________________ Sex M__ F __

Estimated date of confinement ____________________

Date form completed ____________________

Mother's name ________________________________

Mother's hospital number ____________________

Item	Optimal response		Nonoptimal response	
1. Gestational age	>37 wk	☐	<37 wk	☐
2. Birthweight	2,500 gm	☐	<2,500 gm	☐
3. Marital status	Married	☐	Other	☐
4. Maternal age	18–30 yr	☐	Other	☐
5. Previous abortions	2 or fewer	☐	3 or more	☐
6. Previous premature births	No	☐	Yes	☐
7. Previous stillbirths	No	☐	Yes	☐
8. Prolonged unwanted sterility	No	☐	Yes	☐
9. Length of time since last pregnancy	> 12 mo	☐	< 12 mo	☐
10. Parity	1 to 6	☐	0 or $\geq$ 7	☐
11. Pelvis	No disproportion	☐	Disproportion	☐
12. Rh antagonism or other blood-group incompatibility	No	☐	Yes	☐

(continued)

TABLE 2-5. (*Continued*)

Item	Optimal response		Nonoptimal response	
13. Bleeding during pregnancy	No	☐	Yes	☐
14. Infections or other acute medical problems during pregnancy	No	☐	Yes	☐
15. Drugs given to mother during pregnancy	No	☐	Yes	☐
16. Maternal chronic diseases	No	☐	Yes	☐
17. Chronic drug abuse	No	☐	Yes	☐
18. Blood pressure during pregnancy	<140/90	☐	>140/90	☐
19. Albuminuria	No	☐	Yes	☐
20. Hyperemesis	No	☐	Yes	☐
21. Hemoglobin level at end of pregnancy	⩾10	☐	<10	☐
22. Twins or multiple birth	No	☐	Yes	☐
23. Membranes ruptured prior to delivery	0–12 hr	☐	>12 hr	☐
24. Delivery	Spontaneous	☐	Other	☐
25. Forceps	None or elective, low forceps	☐	Other	☐
26. Duration, first stage	3–20 hr	☐	<3 or >20 hr	☐
27. Duration, second stage	10–120 min	☐	<10 or >120 min	☐
28. Induced labor	No	☐	Yes	☐
29. Drugs during labor and delivery	No	☐	Yes	☐
30. Amniotic fluid	Clear	☐	Other	☐
31. Fetal presentation—delivery	Vertex	☐	Other	☐
32. Fetal heart rate during labor	100–160 beats/min	☐	<100 or >160 beats/min	☐
33. Nuchal or knotted cord	No	☐	Yes	☐
34. Cord prolapse	No	☐	Yes	☐
35. Placental infarction	No	☐	Yes	☐
36. Placenta previa or abruptio	No	☐	Yes	☐
37. Onset of stable respiration within 6 min	Yes	☐	No	☐
38. Resuscitation required	No	☐	Yes	☐
39. Prenatal care during first half of pregnancy	Yes	☐	No	☐
40. Apgar score—1 min	7–10	☐	0–6	☐
41. Apgar score—5 min	7–10	☐	0–6	☐

a. Total (raw score)	☐
b. Number of items recorded	☐
c. % raw score (a/b)	☐

Note. Reprinted by permission of Bruce Littman.

score. The total score is divided by the number of items scored, to compensate for any missing data. A conversion table is provided, so that raw scores can be converted to standardized scale scores. No risk category scores are provided.

Littman and Parmelee do not report on the scale's reliability, but its validity was assessed using three scales that they devised: the Postnatal Complications Scale (PNCS) (shown in Table 2-6) and the two Pediatric Complications Scales (PCSs) (shown in Table 2-7). The PNCS is composed of 10 items that describe complications that may arise in an infant in the postnatal period. There are PCSs for infants at 4 months and infants at 9 months. Both PCSs are composed of items related to normal head, weight, and length growth rates; illness, injury, seizure, hospitalizations, feeding difficulties, abnormalities in sleeping, various anomalies, and neurological abnormalities. Conversion tables are provided for both the PNCS and

TABLE 2-6. Littman and Parmelee's (1978) Postnatal Complications Scale

Infant's name ______________________ Sex M __ F __

Hospital number ______________________

Birth date ______________________

Estimated date of confinement ______________________

Date form completed ______________________

Item				
1. Respiratory distress	No	☐	Yes	☐
2. Positive or suspected infection	No	☐	Yes	☐
3. Ventilatory assistance	No	☐	Yes	☐
4. Noninfectious illness or anomaly	No	☐	Yes	☐
5. Metabolic disturbance	No	☐	Yes	☐
6. Convulsion	No	☐	Yes	☐
7. Hyperbilirubinemia or exchange transfusion	No	☐	Yes	☐
8. Temperature disturbance	No	☐	Yes	☐
9. Feeding within 48 hr	No	☐	Yes	☐
10. Surgery	No	☐	Yes	☐
Total (Raw score)		☐		

Note. Reprinted by permission of Bruce Littman.

TABLE 2-7. Littman and Parmelee's (1978) Pediatric Complications Scales—4 Months and 9 Months

Infant's name ______________________ Sex M __ F __

Hospital number ______________________

Birth date ______________________

Estimated date of confinement ______________________

Date form completed ______________________

Item				
1. Head—abnormal rate of growth	No	☐	Yes	☐
2. Weight—abnormal rate of growth	No	☐	Yes	☐
3. Length—abnormal rate of growth	No	☐	Yes	☐
4. Illness occurrence	No	☐	Yes	☐
5. Injury occurrence	No	☐	Yes	☐
6. Seizure	No	☐	Yes	☐
7. Hospitalization (for illness or injury)	No	☐	Yes	☐
8. Hospitalization (for surgery)	No	☐	Yes	☐
9. Persistent feeding difficulty	No	☐	Yes	☐
10. Abnormal crying pattern[a]	No	☐	Yes	☐
11. Abnormal sleeping pattern	No	☐	Yes	☐
12. Craniofacial anomaly	No	☐	Yes	☐
13. Cardiopulmonary anomaly	No	☐	Yes	☐
14. Abdominal anomaly	No	☐	Yes	☐
15. Genitourinary anomaly	No	☐	Yes	☐
16. Extremity anomaly	No	☐	Yes	☐
17. Neurological abnormality of the eyes	No	☐	Yes	☐
18. Neurological abnormality of the face	No	☐	Yes	☐
19. Neurological abnormality of the neck and trunk	No	☐	Yes	☐
20. Neurological abnormality of the extremities	No	☐	Yes	☐
21. Hearing deficit[b]	No	☐	Yes	☐
22. Visual deficit[b]	No	☐	Yes	☐
Total (Raw score)		☐		

Note. Reprinted by permission of Bruce Littman.

[a]"Abnormal activity pattern" on 9-month form.

[b]On 9-month form only.

the PCSs, so that raw scores can be converted to standardized scale scores. The reported correlations between the OCS and the PNCS and between the OCS and PCSs are low (r range = .04 to .28), with high scores related to a greater number of postnatal and pediatric complications.

The Littman and Parmelee validation study was criticized

by Copland (1980) for two methodological problems. First, he pointed out that the only comparison was between summary scores—the score on the OCS versus scores on the PNCS and PCSs. From Copland's point of view, correlations between the summary scores might have been less revealing than correlations between specific items on the OCS and the outcome scales. Second, Coplan noted that the validation study did not differentiate between complications detected in later infancy that were due to antepartum complications and new complications that arose in later infancy. He suggested that interitem correlations between the OCS and the PNCS and PCSs might be useful for revealing the interrelationships between specific types of obstetric complications and specific outcomes during the postnatal and later infancy periods. Littman (1980) responded to these criticisms by noting that the OCS, the PNCS, and the PCSs contained too few items to permit meaningful interitem correlations. Littman also noted that later complications that arose as a result of obstetric complications should have resulted in significant OCS and PCS correlations but that these were not found. Others (e.g., Parmelee & Haber, 1973) have noted that interitem correlations are typically weaker than summary scores and are therefore unlikely to yield useful information.

The OCS has been widely used, especially in conjunction with the Brazelton Neonatal Behavioral Assessment Scale and in studies of neonatal functioning. In most of these studies, the OCS has been used as a system for screening perinatal complications in infants, as a means of describing subject characteristics, or as a predictive tool in studying infant development.

Use of the OCS as a Screening System

Several researchers have incorporated the OCS into their research as a screening system. Widmayer and Field (1980) used the OCS to rule out pregnancy complications as possible intervening variables in a study of the usefulness of the Brazelton neonatal Behavioral Assessment Scale in enhancing mothers' interactions with their preterm infants. Mothers who observed the administration of the Brazelton scale to their infants were more adept after the observation at feeding and interacting with their infants. Anderson (1983) used the OCS to select subjects for a similar study of the enhancement of maternal–infant interactions. Primiparous mothers who observed an administration of the Brazelton scale to their infants and who received an explanation of their infants' performance showed a greater increase in the number of mother–infant interactions. Another intervention study was reported by Field, Widmayer, Stringer, and Ignatoff (1980). These researchers used the OCS, together with demographic measures, measures of infant status (including the PNCS), the Brazelton scale, measures of maternal stress and attitudes, and infant developmental assessment scales, to characterize infants in a study of lower-class black teenage mothers with preterm infants. Overall, the results showed that the infants whose mothers were involved in the intervention program, including those with high OCS scores, generally had better developmental outcomes than the infants of mothers not in the program.

Use of the OCS to Characterize Infants

The OCS has also been used to characterize infants in research studies not related to intervention programs. Field *et al.* (1982) examined the effects on premature infants of nonnutritive sucking during tube feedings. In this study, both the OCS and the PNCS were used to characterize infants. Performance on the Brazelton scale was used as an outcome measure. The infants who were given pacifiers during tube feedings averaged fewer feedings, gained more weight per day, and were discharged earlier than control infants, who were not given pacifiers. Their performance on the Brazelton scale, however, was poorer than that of the control group. In another study, Field, Sandberg, Quetel, Garcia, and Rosario (1985) used the OCS to characterize women who received video and verbal feedback while undergoing ultrasound examinations. Compared to a control group of women who did not receive such feedback, those who received the feedback had fewer obstetric complications and produced neonates who had heavier and more appropriate-for-their-length birthweights, who were less active and irritable, and who performed better on the Brazelton scale. Woodson (1987) used the OCS and the PNCS to characterize 110 low-risk infants in a study of behavioral and biochemical stability during the first 3 days of life. Behavior, as measured by the Brazelton scale, was found to be unreliable across times of measurement but reliably related to the biochemical measures.

The OCS scores have been less frequently used to characterize subjects in studies that have not also used the Brazelton scale. One of these few is a study by Zeskind and Iacinco (1984), who examined the effect of mothers' visits to a neonatal intensive care unit on the subsequent interactions of the mothers with their preterm infants. The items on the OCS pertaining to infants were used to assess the infants and to assign them to experimental or control groups.

Use of the OCS as a Predictive Tool

In other studies, the OCS has been used as a predictive tool. Interestingly, this scale was found not to be a significant predictor of the various outcome measures used in most of these studies. For example, Rose *et al.* (1980) studied cardiac and behavioral responsivity of full-term and preterm infants during sleep. Risk factors included such measures as birthweight, gestational age, and scores on both the OCS and the PNCS. Only birthweight and gestational age were found to be significant correlates of cardiac and behavioral responsivity. Cohen, Parmelee, Sigman, and Beckwith (1982) used the OCS in a longitudinal (birth to 5 years) study of 59 premature infants. They found that prenatal and postnatal medical complications as measured by the OCS and the PNCS were not significantly related to performance in later infancy and childhood on the Bayley Scales of Infant Development, the Gesell Developmental Schedules, and the Stanford–Binet. However, all the children who performed poorly at age 5 had had neonatal complications. The authors pointed to the caretaking environment as an important component in modifying and supporting cognitive development. Cohen, Sigman, Parmelee, and Beckwith (1982) reported on a study in which the OCS was used to characterize and evaluate a sample of premature infants. They found that OCS scores were not significantly related to scores on the Gesell Developmental Schedules and on the Stanford–Binet in later infancy. Similar findings were reported by Reich, Holmes, Slaymaker, Lauesen, and Gyurke (1984) in a study of 52 infants that was designed to identify predictors of performance on an intelligence test at 3 years of age. The study sample was composed of preterm infants, full-term infants in intensive care, full-term infants with sick mothers, and healthy full-term infants. Data were obtained at birth on the OCS, the PNCS, and the Brazelton scale; at age 18 months on the Bayley—Mental Scale and the Bayley—Motor Scale; and at 36 months on the Stanford–Binet. Scores on the Bayley scales were the only significant predictors of the Stanford–Binet scores.

In two studies, the OCS was found to be a significant predictor of infant behaviors. Holmes, Ruble, Kowalski, and Lauesen (1984) reported that amount of neonatal crying and OCS scores were predictive of anxious versus secure attachments in 24 who were 1 year of age. Other variables (e.g., 1-minute Apgar scores, Brazelton Interactive Processes scores, and sex) were also predictive but were weaker than the measures of amount of crying and OCS scores. Mothers of anxiously attached children had had more intrapartum complications than had mothers of securely attached children. Salter, Holmes, Reich, and Slaymaker (1987) used a modified version of the OCS in a study of maternal attitudes and expectations. The researchers modified the OCS by using the antepartum items only and by adding items related to substance abuse and major life stress events. In their prospective sample of 27 women, perinatal risk scores were significantly correlated at birth with birthweight (r = .67), maternal perception of the "average baby" (r = .39) and maternal self-perception scores (r = 37), and at 2 weeks postpartum with maternal perception of their own infants (r = .57). The perinatal risk scores were not significantly correlated with other postpartum perception measures.

The PNCS alone has been examined in several studies. For example, Wrate, Rooney, Thomas, and Cox (1985) studied the relationship between maternal postnatal depression and behavioral disturbances in children. In a sample of 91 mothers and their children, the researchers found that scores on the PNCS were not associated with childhood behavioral disturbances, although episodes of postnatal depression were related to childhood disturbances.

MATERNAL–CHILD HEALTH CARE INDEX

The Maternal–Child Health Care Index (MCHCI) (Nesbitt & Aubry, 1969) is based on a scoring system in which 100 is a perfect score. Conditions presumed to negatively influence perinatal outcome are assigned a penalty score that is weighted to estimate the degree of risk. The MCHCI (shown in Table 2-8) contains six categories of antepartum items, an emotional survey category, and a socioeconomic survey category. The items in the six categories pertain to maternal age, race, marital status, parity, past obstetric history, medical–obstetric disorders, nutrition, and generative tract disorders. The emotional survey covers such aspects as fear, attitudes, and marital relationship and the socioeconomic survey, such factors as employment, and education.

Aubry and Pennington (1973) later introduced the Labor Index (LI) for use with the MCHCI. The LI (shown in Table 2-9) contains 14 intrapartum items grouped into three categories: maternal, placental, and fetal. There are no items pertaining to the postnatal status of the infant.

The items on the MCHCI are assigned weights of 0, 5, 10, 15, 20, or 30, and items on the LI are assigned weights of 10, 20, or 30. Scores on the MCHCI and the LI can be summed to obtain a total score. Risk categories for the MCHCI are assigned as follows: "low risk" = 85 points and over; "moderate risk" = 70 to 84 points; "high risk" = 69 points and under. Comparable categories for the LI have not been detailed.

Nesbitt and Aubry (1969) reported on the validity of the MCHCI in a study of 1,001 consecutive patients who were screened for perinatal risk during their initial prenatal visit. Infants of patients with low scores on the MCHCI (i.e., "high-risk" patients) were found to have had poorer outcomes as measured by low birthweight, preterm birth, infection, birth

TABLE 2-8. Nesbitt and Aubry's (1969) Maternal–Child Health Care Index

Name: ______________ Date: ______________ EDC: ______________ Hospital: ______________
& Number: ______________

The scoring system below is an attempt to categorize the degree of maternal and fetal risk based on the information available at the initial history and physical upon registration in our obstetric clinics. Please circle the numbers under each of the 8 categories that you feel apply and, at the bottom of this sheet, add up these numbers and subtract from a perfect score of 100.

I. Maternal age		II. Race and marital status		III. Parity	
Under 15 yr	20	White	0	0	10
15–19 yr	10	Nonwhite	5	1–3	0
20–29 yr	0	Single	5	4–7	5
30–34 yr	5	Married	0	Over 8	10
35–39 yr	10				
Over 40 yr	20				

IV. Past obstetric history

Abortions		*Premature births*		*Fetal deaths*		*Neonatal deaths*		*Congenital anomalies*		*Damaged infants*	
1	5	1	10	1	10	1	10	1	10	Physical	10
2	15	2+	20	2+	30	2+	30	2+	20	Neurological	20
3+	30										

V. Medical–obstetric disorders and nutrition

Systemic illnesses		*Specific infections*		*Diabetes*		*Chronic hypertension*	
Acute, mild	5	Urinary		Prediabetes	20	Mild	15
Acute, serious	15	Acute	5	Overt	30	Severe	30
Chronic, nondebilitating	5	Chronic	25			Nephritis	30
Chronic, debilitating	20	Syphilis					
		Treated	0			*Heart disease*	
		Untreated	20			Class I or II	10
		At term	30			Class III or IV	30
						History of prior failure	30

Endocrine disorders		*Anemia*	
Definite adrenal, pituitary, or thyroid problem	30	Hb, 10–11 gm	5
Recurrent menstrual dysfunction	10	Hb, 9–10 gm	10
Involuntary sterility		Hb, less than 9 gm	20
Less than 2 yr	10		
More than 2 yr	20		

Rh problem		*Nutrition*	
Sensitized	30	Malnourished	20
Prior infant affected	30	Very obese	30
Prior ABO incompatibility	20	Inadequate diet but not malnourished	10

(continued)

TABLE 2-8. *(Continued)*

VI.	Generative tract disorders		VII.	Emotional survey—Grade 0–20 based on:
	Prior fetal malpresentations	10		Fears, attitudes, biases, hostilities, motivations, and behavioral patterns; prior pregnancies without supervision; time of registration; standard of child care and responsibilities; family unit, marital relationship; history of psychiatric illness in family.
	Prior cesarean section	30		
	Known anomaly or incompetent cervix	20		
	Myomas			
	Over 5 cm	20		
	Submucous	30		
	Contracted pelvis			
	Borderline	10		
	Any contracted plane	30		
	Ovarian masses			
	Over 6 cm	20		
	Endometriosis	5		
VIII.	Social and economic survey—Grade 0–10 based on:			
	Employment—husband, patient; annual income adequacy; public assistance			
	Education—husband, patient			
	Housing—location, quality, facilities, and neighborhood environment			
Total score of all 8 categories		______		
100 less above score equals MCHCI		______		

Note. From "High-Risk Obstetrics" by R. E. Nesbitt, Jr., and R. H. Aubry, 1969. *American Journal of Obstetrics and Gynecology, 103*, p. 972. Copyright 1969 by C. V. Mosby Co. Reprinted by permission.

TABLE 2-9. Aubry and Pennington's (1973) Labor Index

Factors	Penalty points
Maternal factors	
1. Prenatal care	
<3 prenatal visits	10
No prenatal visits	20
2. Toxemia	
Mild	20
Severe	30
3. Undetected diabetes	20
4. Anemia—Hb <10 gm	10
5. Fever	20
Placental factors	
1. Bleeding before 20 wk	10
2. Bleeding 20 wk–term	20
3. Bleeding with pain and/or hypotension	30
4. Ruptured membranes >24 hr	20
Fetal factors	
1. Gestational age	
< 34 wk	30
34–37 wk	20
> 42 wk	20
2. Multiple pregnancy	20
3. Previously undetected Rh sensitization	20
4. Meconium staining	30
5. Fetal heart rate abnormality (<115, >165)	30
Labor Index score = 100 − above penalties	
Total Index = 200 − (penalties from MCHCI and penalties from Labor Index)	

Note. MCHCI = Maternal–Child Health Care Index. From "Identification and Evaluation of High-Risk Pregnancy: The Perinatal Concept" by R. Aubry and J. Pennington, 1973. *Clinical Obstetrics and Gynecology, 16,* p. 9. Copyright 1973 by Harper & Row. Reprinted by permission.

injury, respiratory distress, low Apgar scores, mortality, and such maternal complications as toxemia, placental problems, labor complications, and incidence of cesarean section. No reliability estimates were reported.

Jones (1978) used a modified version of the MCHCI in a study of 122 pregnant women who were described as "essentially healthy." Pregnancy complications, measures of anxiety, life changes, and personality variables were used as predictors of labor complications. It was found that life-change scores were the only ones that discriminated between women with labor complications and those without such complications. Surprisingly, women with low life-change scores experienced more complications. The author described the sample as having a high overall level of life changes. In this sample, "low" life-change scores are equivalent to moderate- and high-level scores in other samples. The results do seem to confirm the belief that a greater number of life changes has a negative influence on intrapartum events.

The MCHCI was also used in a study of women with psychiatric disorders that was conducted by Powers, Johnson, Knuppel, Cupoli, and Achenback (1986). Fifty women who were identified as "high risk" based on the MCHCI were also assessed for psychiatric disorders. Of these women, only 18 were found to be without significant psychiatric disorders. The authors concluded that because these patients were drawn from a lower socioeconomic population, they were at greater risk for psychiatric disorders as well as for chronic physical and physiological disorders. Because these women were also found to have rather negative attitudes toward pregnancy as measured by the Maternal Attitude to Pregnancy Instrument (Blau, Welkowitz, & Cohen, 1964), the authors cautioned that they needed special prenatal care.

Aubry and Pennington (1973) examined the validity of the MCHCI and the LI with approximately 450 consecutive patients who were admitted to the labor and delivery unit of Upstate Medical Center, Syracuse, New York. Infants of patients with low scores on both the MCHCI and the LI had the highest risks of poor outcomes (e.g., prematurity, low birthweight, neonatal depression, and respiratory distress syndrome), followed by infants of patients with low scores on the LI and then by infants of patients with low MCHCI scores. The MCHCI alone predicted 52% of the perinatal deaths, and the LI alone predicted an additional 30%. It is interesting to note that the intrapartum scores were more accurate in predicting morbidity than were the antepartum scores. This finding is similar to that reported by Hobel *et al.* (1973).

SCALE OF OPTIMAL OBSTETRIC CONDITIONS

Prechtl's Scale of Optimal Obstetric Conditions (OOC) was developed by Prechtl (1967) based on the results of a study of

1,378 full-term neonates. Data based on Prechtl and Beintema's (1964) Neurological Examination of the Full-Term Newborn Infant and data pertaining to pregnancy, delivery, and postnatal status were obtained from these infants. The resultant scale (shown in Table 2-10) is composed of 42 items grouped into three categories: maternal factors (20 items), parturition (8 items), and fetal factors (14 items). Characteristics that do not deviate from optimal conditions are given 0 points, whereas those that do are given 1 point. The presence of 0 to 1 nonoptimal conditions is considered "low risk," 2 to 6 nonoptimal

TABLE 2-10. Prechtl's (1968) Criteria of Optimal Obstetric Conditions

Maternal factors	
1. Maternal age primipara	18–30 yr
Maternal age multipara	20–30 yr
2. Marital state	Married
3. Parity	1–6
4. Abortions in history	0–2
5. Pelvis	No disproportion
6. Luetic infection	Absent
7. Rh antagonism	Absent
8. Blood-group incompatibility	Absent
9. Nutritional state	Well nourished
10. Hemoglobin level	70 or more
11. Bleeding during pregnancy	Absent
12. Infections during pregnancy	Absent
13. X-ray abdomen during pregnancy	No
14. Toxemia	Absent or mild
15. Blood pressure	Not exceeding 90/135
16. Albuminuria and edema	Absent
17. Hyperemesis	Absent
18. Psychological stress	Absent
19. Prolonged unwanted sterility (2 yr)	Absent
20. Maternal chronic diseases	Absent
Parturition	
21. Twins or multiple birth	No
22. Delivery	Spontaneous
23. Duration 1st-stage labor	6–24 hr
24. Duration 2nd-stage labor	10 min–2 hr
25. Contractions	Moderate or strong
26. Drugs given to mother	Oxygen, local anesthetic
27. Amniotic fluid	Clear
28. Membranes broken	Not longer than 6 hr

(*continued*)

TABLE 2-10. *(Continued)*

Fetal factors	
29. Intrauterine position	Vertex
30. Gestational age	38–41 wk
31. Fetal presentation	Vertex
32. Cardiac regularity	Regular
33. Fetal heart rate (2nd-stage labor)	100–160 beats per min
34. Cord around the neck	No or loose
35. Cord prolapse	No
36. Knot in the cord	No
37. Placental infarction	No or small
38. Onset respiration	Within 1 min
39. Treatment, resuscitation	No
40. Drugs given	No
41. Body temperature	Normal
42. Birthweight	2,500–4,990 gm

Note. From "Neurological Findings in Newborn Infants after Pre- and Paranatal Complications" by H. F. R. Prechtl, 1968. In J. Jonxis, H. Vissern, and J. Trodstran (Eds.), *Aspects of Prematurity and Dysmaturity: Nutricia Symposium,* pp. 306–307. Springfield, IL: Charles C Thomas. Copyright 1968 by Charles C Thomas. Reprinted by permission.

conditions "medium risk," and 7 or more nonoptimal conditions "high risk."

Reliability of the OOC has not been reported, but validity has been assessed in several different studies. In early research reports by Prechtl (1967, 1968), the validity of the scale was established using Prechtl and Beintema's (1964) Neurological Examination of the Full-Term Newborn Infant and a variety of perinatal measures. High scores on the OOC (indicative of high risk) were found to be associated with higher incidences of neurological abnormalities (apathy syndrome, hypotonia). High scores on the OOC were also found to be associated with higher incidences of toxemia, cesarean section, use of forceps, fetal distress, and apnea of less than 1 minute (Prechtl, 1967, 1968).

Several studies have examined the relationship between OOC scores and neurological development in infants and children. Forslund and Bjerre (1983), who studied 46 premature infants, found a nonsignificant relationship between OOC scores and neurological development. Remo, Largo, and Pfister (1987) conducted a longitudinal study of 95 children and a cross-sectional study of 249 children, all of whom were between the ages of 5 and 7 years. Perinatal risk scores from the OOC, plus scores on 51 items added by the authors, were used to evaluate language, cognitive, and neurological development. The perinatal scores were reported to show "low positive, [and] inconsistently significant correlations" with the outcome measures. The perinatal scores were described as "only of minor significance" compared to socioeconomic status and minor physical malformations scores.

Sepkoski *et al.* (1977) used a modification of the OOC in a study of 121 normal newborns. Predictions of performance scores on the four *a priori* dimensions and on the overall profile of the Brazelton Neonatal Behavioral Assessment Scale were made on the basis of the OOC scores. High nonoptimal scores on the OOC Maternal subscale were significantly associated with low scores on the Brazelton Interactive Processes, Physiological Response to Stress, and overall scale profile. High nonoptimal scores on the OOC Parturition subscale were significantly associated with low scores on Motoric Processes, State Control, and Physiological Response to Stress. High nonoptimal scores on the Fetal subscale were significantly associated with low scores on Motoric Processes and Physiological Response to Stress. Combinations of OOC scores with other variables (birthweight, hospitalization, length of labor, type of delivery, sex of infant, ponderal index, and gestational age) contributed to the significant prediction of performance on the four dimensions and overall profile of the Brazelton scale.

ROCHESTER RESEARCH OBSTETRICAL SCALE

The Rochester Research Obstetrical Scale (RROS) was developed by Zax *et al.* (1977) from versions of the Prechtl OOC (1967) that were revised for U.S. populations by Parmelee (Beckwith, Cohen, & Parmelee, 1973). Norms for the RROS were obtained from data on 40,000 pregnancies as reported by the National Institute of Neurological Diseases and Stroke collaborative study (Niswander & Gordon, 1972). The RROS (shown in Table 2-11) contains 27 items grouped into three categories: prenatal (6 items), delivery (13 items), and infant (8 items). Each item is assigned a weight from 1 to 4, and item

TABLE 2-11. Zax, Sameroff, and Babigian's (1977) Rochester Research Obstetrical Scale

Prenatal scale

1. Young mother (primigravida < 16 years, multigravida <18)
2. Old mother (>35 years)
3. Grand multiparity (> 6)
4. Abortions (> 2)
5. Chronic medication (excluding vitamins)
6. Physical disorders (chronic disease or infections, 1 point each up to 4 points)

Delivery scale

7. Cesarean section (planned = 1 point, unplanned = 2 points)
8. Induction
9. Premature rupture of membranes
10. Presentation (not vertex)
11. Cord (knotted, prolapsed, or tight around neck)
12. Placenta problem
13. Amniotic fluid (turbid = 1 point, bloody = 2 points)
14. Multiple gestation
15. Forceps (low = 1 point, mid or high = 2 points)
16. Analgesia (> 50 mg = 1 point, > 100 mg = 2 points)
17. Anesthesia (> local or pudendal block = 1 point, general = 2 points)
18. Long labor
    (primigravida: stage I > 20 hr or stage II > 2 hr)
    (multigravida: stage I > 20 hr or stage II > 2 hr)
19. Short labor
    (primigravida: stage I < 3 hr or stage II < 10 min)
    (multigravida: stage I < 2 hr or stage II < 10 min)

Infant scale

20. Low birthweight (< 2,500 gm) and/or premature birth
21. Low fetal heart rate (2 points)
22. Neonatal heart rate < 100
23. Resuscitation necessary
24. 5-min Apgar < 8
25. Gross physical anomaly (2 points)
26. Fetal or neonatal death (< 30 days) (3 points)
27. Physical disorders (1 point each up to 3 points)

Note. Total score = sum of prenatal, delivery, and infant scores. Each item scores 1 point unless otherwise indicated. From "Early Development of Children at Risk for Emotional Disorder" by A. Sameroff, R. Seifer, and M. Zax, 1982. *Monographs of the Society for Research in Child Development, 47*, p. 22. Copyright 1982 by the Society for Research in Child Development. Reprinted by permission.

scores can be summed to obtain a total scale score or subscale scores. No risk category scores are provided.

The validity of the scale has been assessed in two studies of normal and mentally ill women (Zax *et al.,* 1977; Sameroff, Seifer, & Zax, 1982), one of which utilized a large longitudinal sample (Sameroff *et al.,* 1982). In both studies, mental health diagnosis, severity of symptomatology, and chronicity of illness were predictive of RROS Delivery and Infant scores. In addition, although specific statistical results were not reported, high RROS scores appear to relate to lower 1- and 5-minute Apgar scores, lower birthweight, higher incidence of resuscitation and fetal deaths, and poorer scores on the Rochester Adaptive Behavior Inventory (RABI) (Seifer, Sameroff, & Jones, 1981). Correlations between Delivery subscale scores and RABI scores are .14. Reliability estimates for the scale have not been reported.

Firestone and Prabhu (1983) used a revision of the RROS in a study of 52 boys aged 5 to 12 years. The boys were classified as hyperactive, psychoneurotic, or normal. Measures of minor physical anomalies and RROS scores, based on mothers' reports, were used as the dependent variables. The hyperactive boys, in contrast to the psychoneurotic and normal (control) boys, were more often characterized as having a large number of minor physical anomalies and perinatal complications.

Marcus, Auerback, Wilkinson, and Burack (1981) used the RROS to assess antepartum, perinatal, and postpartum risks in a sample of 54 parents, 17 of whom were diagnosed as schizophrenic, 6 as having affective disorders, 13 as having personality disorders and 18 as normal. No group differences were found on the RROS. However, infants of the schizophrenic parents, compared to infants of the other parents, were found to show poor motor and sensorimotor performance on the Brazelton scale at birth and on the Bayley scales during the first year of life. Perinatal risk scores on the RROS were not predictive of parental diagnoses for infants of schizophrenic parents.

The RROS has been used by other researchers primarily to characterize subjects in their studies rather than as a predictive tool. Green (1984) used the scale to characterize perinatal risk in samples of schizophrenic, autistic, and conduct-disordered children. It was found that the mothers of conduct-disordered children had used more illegal and nonprescription drugs during pregnancy than the mothers of schizophrenic and autistic children. Jeremy and Bernstein (1984) used the RROS to characterize 42 women of lower socioeconomic status aged 18 to 34 years, 18 of whom were being maintained on methadone and 24 who were not. Methadone dosage in pregnancy, length of opioid use, RROS scores, birthweight, and gestational age were found not to be predictive of communicative functioning and performance on the measures of maternal psychological and psychosocial resources and infant motor development as assessed on the Bayley Scales of Infant Development (Bayley, 1969). Poor maternal resources in the mothers and poor motor functioning in the infants were predictive of mother–infant dyadic interactions.

SUMMARY

The six perinatal risk scales described in this chapter have been used in various research and clinical studies. Although no validity data have been published on the Brazie *et al.* UCNM and few data have been published on the MCHCI (Nesbitt & Aubry) and the LI (Aubry & Pennington), the validity of the other scales has been examined in a wide variety of studies. The scales developed by Hobel *et al.* (the HRPSS), Littman and Parmelee (the OCS), Prechtl (the OOC), and Zax, Sameroff, and Babigian (the RROS) have generally all been shown to be valid predictors of perinatal outcomes. Extensions of the scales to predict behaviors during infancy and childhood have produced more inconsistent and negative results. Direct comparisons of the accuracy of two or more of the scales in predicting various outcomes have not been reported in the literature independent of the work reported by Molfese and colleagues (Molfese & Thomson, 1985; Molfese *et al.*, 1985; Molfese, Thomson, *et al.*, 1987). Such direct comparisons are needed in order to determine whether one perinatal risk scale is as good as another in predicting outcomes during the perinatal period and during later infancy and childhood.

CHAPTER

3

The Predictive Values of Perinatal Risk Scales

In the previous chapter, six perinatal risk scales were described and examples given of their use in research and clinical settings. Although these scales have been shown to be useful for a variety of research and clinical purposes, there have been few studies in which the screening performance of one scale has been directly compared to the performance of other scales in predicting outcome measures. Such comparisons are important because the results would provide a basis for scale selection that is currently unavailable. If one scale could be identified as being better than other scales in predicting all outcomes or specific types of outcomes, the task of scale selection would be simplified. This chapter describes a research project (Molfese *et al.,* 1985) that focused on the question, Are the scores generated by the various perinatal risk scales equally useful in predicting measures of the postnatal status of mothers and their infants?

The perinatal risk scales are used to provide information on three issues of importance to scale selection. The first issue is whether one scale is as good as another in screening obstetric patients or research subjects for perinatal risk. By examining both the similarity of a subject's risk scores across scales and the contribution of these scores in predictive models of perinatal outcome, this issue can be addressed. The second issue is one that was raised by Hobel *et al.* (1973) concerning the predictive value of intrapartum risk scores versus that of antepartum risk scores. Hobel *et al.* (1973) reported that intrapartum scores are more accurate predictors of maternal and infant outcomes than are antepartum scores. Support for this finding has also been provided by others (Sokol *et al.,* 1977; Nesbitt & Aubry, 1969). By examining the contribution made by intrapartum scores versus that made by antepartum scores to the prediction of specific outcome measures, this finding can be verified. The third issue is whether number of complications as a measure of perinatal risk is a more valid predictor of infant outcome than are scores calculated from risk scales. This issue was raised by Strobino and Baruffi (1984), who reported that number of complications is both easier to calculate and more accurate in predicting outcome than are actual risk scores. Prechtl (1967) has claimed that a simple count of the number of risk conditions is a useful measure of perinatal risk. This issue can be addressed by comparing the magnitude of correlations between actual risk scores and outcome measures with the magnitude of correlations between number of complications and outcome measures.

In the Molfese *et al.* (1985) research project, five of the six perinatal risk scales described in Chapter 2 were evaluated. The scale developed by Prechtl (1967) was not included because of its similarity to the Littman and Parmelee (1978) scale, which was evaluated under the project. A separate study that examined the predictive validity of the Prechtl scale in comparison with some of the other scales is described in Chapter 4.

DESCRIPTION OF THE STUDY

Data were obtained in a retrospective study (Molfese *et al.,* 1985) of 116 postpartum women and their infants. These subjects were randomly selected from a sample of women who participated in a study of routine fetal monitoring. The women in this sample ranged in age from 15 to 38 years ($\bar{x}$ = 24.9 years). All of the women delivered live infants, 18 by cesarean section. The infants' birthweights ranged from 1,559 to 5,046 grams ($\bar{x}$ = 3,478 grams), and the infants ranged in gestational age from 31 to 44 weeks ($\bar{x}$ = 39.8 weeks). The average 1- and 5-minute Apgar scores were 7.69 (range = 1 to 9) and 8.72 (range = 4 to 10), respectively. Nine of the infants were preterm and were placed in special care nurseries. Other demographic information that was used to score scale items is given in Table 3-1.

During the postpartum period, scores were obtained for each of the five scales being evaluated. Each scale was scored directly from demographic information forms completed by the women and from the information contained in their medical records. Information relevant to the antepartum period was taken from antepartum medical records; intrapartum information, from labor and delivery records; and postpartum information, from postpartum and nursery records that noted the condition of the mother and the infant until discharge. Because the hospital medical records were kept on standardized forms and contain detailed information, scoring problems due to missing or incomplete data were minimized. In each

TABLE 3-1. Demographic Characteristics of the Study Sample of 116 Women

Marital status		Parity		Income	
Single	16	0 births	55	Under $5,000	2
Married	100	1–4 births	60	$5,000–10,000	6
		5 or more births	1	$10,000–15,000	21
				$15,000–20,000	18
				$20,000–25,000	24
				$25,000–30,000	15
				$30,000–35,000	21
				Over $35,000	2
				No information	7

Education—wife		Education—husband	
Less than high school graduate	16	Less than high school graduate	18
High school graduate	11	High school graduate	14
Some college	35	Some college	25
College graduate	42	College graduate	36
Postgraduate	12	Postgraduate	7
		No information	16

Employment—wife		Employment—husband	
Employed	48	Employed	95
Unemployed	68	Unemployed	6
		No information	15

case, scores were obtained using the exact parameters specified by each scale. Scales were initially scored by two coders and checked for accuracy by an additional coder.

Descriptive statistics on the five scales are as follows: the University of Colorado Neonatal Morbidity Risk Scale (UCNM) (Brazie *et al.,* cited in Lubchenco, 1976)—mean = 30.24, *SD* = 22.75, range = 9 to 114; the High-Risk Pregnancy Screening System (HRPSS) (Hobel *et al.,* 1973)—mean = 11.68, *SD* = 14.61, range = 0 to 70; the Obstetrical Complications Scale (OCS) (Littman & Parmelee, 1978)—mean = 3.75, *SD* = 2.36, range = 0 to 12; the Maternal–Child Health Care Index (MCHCI) and Labor Index (LI) (Nesbitt & Aubry, 1969; Aubry & Pennington, 1973)—mean = 43.5, *SD* = 27.7, range = 7 to 188; the Rochester Research Obstetrical Scale (RROS) (Zax *et al.,* 1977)—mean = 2.3, *SD* = 2.39, range = 0 to 11.

Both infant and maternal outcome measures were used to evaluate the predictions of the scales. The specific measures used were selected because all of them are measures of morbidity that have been commonly used in reported studies and because many of these measures have been used in the validity studies by developers of these and other perinatal risk scales (Akhtar & Sehgal, 1980; Aubry & Pennington, 1973; Hobel *et al.,* 1973; Morrison *et al.,* 1980; Nesbitt & Aubry, 1969; Ryan *et al.,* 1980; Sokol *et al.,* 1977). The infant outcome measures used were 1- and 5-minute Apgar scores, gestational age, birthweight, respiratory distress syndrome, and each scale's own group of neonatal items, except for the MCHCI + LI, which does not have its own neonatal items. In later analyses involving this scale, the Neonatal subscale from the HRPSS was used because it contains the most extensive array of neonatal items and has been shown in other research to be a valid measure of neonatal morbidity (Strobino & Baruffi, 1984). Primary cesarean section and midforceps delivery were used as maternal outcome measures because they had been used in prior validity studies with some of these scales and because the frequency of these complications is typically high enough to ensure that enough data would be obtained for use in a study of predictive validity.

RESULTS OF THE STUDY

The data were analyzed in several different ways in order to address the three issues raised earlier in the chapter concerning the comparability of risk predictions across scales.

Relative Effectiveness of Scales in Screening for Perinatal Risk

To address the first research issue—that is, the similarity of the subjects' risk scores across scales—Pearson product–moment correlations were computed. Correlations were first computed on total scale scores. The correlation coefficients, shown in Table 3-2, range from .57 to .84 and thus are quite high. These correlations can be interpreted as indicating that the total scores generated by the five scales are generally similar to each other. However, there are markedly lower correlations between the MCHCI + LI and the other four scales, ranging from .57 to .67. These correlations are lower than the other correlations shown in the table, which are all in the .70s and .80s. These low correlations reflect differences in the total risk scores generated by this scale compared to those generated by the other scales.

To explore the source of the differences found for total risk scores, these scores were subsequently divided into an-

Table 3-2. Correlation Coefficients for Total Scale Scores

Scale	RROS	OCS	HRPSS	MCHCI + LI	UCNM
RROS	×				
OCS	.81	×			
HRPSS	.84	.74	×		
MCHCI + LI	.57	.61	.67	×	
UCNM	.71	.70	.74	.60	×

Note. All correlations over .25 are significant ($p < .01$). Abbreviations for scales in this and subsequent tables: RROS = Rochester Research Obstetrical Scale; OCS = Obstetrical Complications Scale; HRPSS = High-Risk Pregnancy Screening System; MCHCI + LI = Maternal–Child Health Care Index and Labor Index; UCNM = University of Colorado Neonatal Morbidity Risk Scale. From "Perinatal Outcome: The Similarity and Predictive Values of Antepartum and Intrapartum Assessment Scales" by V. J. Molfese, B. Thomson, and A. Bennett, 1985. *Journal of Reproductive Medicine, 30,* p. 36. Copyright 1985 by the *Journal of Reproductive Medicine.* Reprinted by permission.

tepartum and intrapartum subscale scores. Pearson product–moment correlations were computed on the subscale scores. The correlation coefficients are shown in Tables 3-3 and 3-4. The antepartum subscale correlations range from .11 to .63. The intrapartum subscale correlations range from .29 to .85. As can be seen, the magnitudes of the correlations on the two subscales are quite variable. The antepartum subscale correlations are for the most part very low, indicating that the antepartum scores that were generated for each subject by the five perinatal risk scales are quite different. The intrapartum subscale correlations are more similar to each other, reflecting the greater similarity in the intrapartum scores generated for each subject by the scales.

The differences in the magnitudes of the correlation coefficients across scales and subscales are hypothesized as having two causes. First, the specific antepartum and intrapartum items included on the scales are not homogeneous. The homogeneity of the scales can be examined by grouping all of the antepartum and intrapartum items contained on the five scales into categories of perinatal conditions. In all, the scales contain 195 different items. With these 195 items, it is possible to construct 23 antepartum and 12 intrapartum categories of perinatal conditions. Each category is composed of items that represent similar conditions that are present on two or more scales. The distribution of scale items within the antepartum and intrapartum categories and the risk definitions of the items included are shown in Tables 3-5 and 3-6.

TABLE 3-3. Correlation Coefficients for Antepartum Subscale Scores

Scale	RROS	OCS	HRPSS	MCHCI + LI	UCNM
RROS	×				
OCS	.45	×			
HRPSS	.37	.32	×		
MCHCI + LI	.30	.34	.63	×	
UCNM	.11	.17	.38	.49	×

Note. All correlations over .25 are significant ($p < .01$). From "Perinatal Outcome: The Similarity and Predictive Values of Antepartum and Intrapartum Assessment Scales" by V. J. Molfese, B. Thomson, and A. Bennett, 1985. *Journal of Reproductive Medicine, 30,* p. 37. Copyright 1985 by the *Journal of Reproductive Medicine.* Reprinted by permission.

TABLE 3-4. Correlation Coefficients for Intrapartum Subscale Scores

Scale	RROS	OCS	HRPSS	MCHCI + LI	UCNM
RROS	×				
OCS	.85	×			
HRPSS	.82	.76	×		
MCHCI + LI	.37	.45	.47	×	
UCNM	.73	.65	.72	.29	×

Note. All correlations over .25 are significant ($p < .01$). From "Perinatal Outcome: The Similarity and Predictive Values of Antepartum and Intrapartum Assessment Scales" by V. J. Molfese, B. Thomson, and A. Bennett, 1985. *Journal of Reproductive Medicine, 30,* p. 37. Copyright 1985 by the *Journal of Reproductive Medicine.* Reprinted by permission.

These categories permit the Pearson product–moment correlations to be viewed from a different perspective. In all cases, the highest correlations occur between those scales that have items that come from the greatest number of similar categories. For example, the highest antepartum correlation is .63, which occurs between the HRPSS and the MCHCI + LI. The items on HRPSS are distributed across 91% of all the antepartum categories in Table 3-5, and the MCHCI + LI items, across 87% of these antepartum categories. Although each of these two scales contains a different number of items, the categories represented by the items on each scale are quite similar. Fewer of the items contained in the other scales are similarly distributed across the categories, as shown by the much lower percentages of distribution across the antepartum categories (i.e., 39%, 61%, and 23% for the UCNM, the OCS, and the RROS, respectively). The lower antepartum correlation coefficients shown by these other scales seem to reflect the dissimilarity of the antepartum items contained on the scales.

With regard to the intrapartum categories, a disparately low 33% of the items on the MCHCI + LI correspond to the intrapartum categories (compared to 63%, for the UCNM and 100% for the HRPSS, the OCS, and the RROS). As shown in Table 3-4, the lowest intrapartum correlations are between the MCHCI + LI and the other four scales. Overall, the generally higher correlations found for the intrapartum subscales as

TABLE 3-5. Antepartum Categories and Risk Definitions from Perinatal Risk Scales

Scale	Abortion	Age	Anemia	Anomaly (prior)	Birthweight (prior infants)	Bleeding	Chronic drug abuse	Drugs in pregnancy	Diabetes
RROS	R = >2	R = <16 yr primigravida = <18 yr multigravida >35 yr						R = Chronic medication	
OCS	R = ⩾3	R = <18 yr >30 yr	R = <10 gm Hb			R = Yes	R = Yes	R = Yes	
HRPSS	R = Habitual abortion	R = <15 yr ⩾35 yr	R = 9–10.9 gm Hb	R = Yes	R = > 10 lb	R = Spotting	R = Yes	R = Smoke ⩾ 1 pack/day; alcohol (moderate use)	R = Family history, types
MCHCI + LI	R = ⩾1	R = <15 yr <20 yr >30 yr	R = <11 gm Hb	R = ⩾1		R = <20 wk >20 wk with pain/ hypotension			R = Undetected or prediabetic or overt
UCNM		R = <17 yr >30 yr			R = low				R = Yes

Scale	Chronic disorders/ diseases	Fertility problems	Gyn. problems	Heart disease	Parity	Prenatal care	Premature infant (prior)	Rh problems (prior)
RROS	R = Chronic diseases or infections				R = >6			
OCS	R = Yes	R = Unwanted sterility	R = Specific problems		R = 0 >7	R = Not in 1st half of pregnancy	R = Yes	R = Antagonism or incompatibility

HRPSS	R = Specific disorders or diseases		R = Specific problems	R = Specific types	R = >5		R = Yes	R = Sensitization or prior infant affected
MCHCI + LI	R = Debilitating or nondebilitating	R = In-voluntary sterility	R = Specific problems	R = Specific classes	R = >0 >4	R = <3 visits	R = ⩾1	R = Previously un-detected sensitization or sensitized, prior infant affected; prior infant incompatibility
UCNM			R = Specific problems			R = 0 visits 1–3 4–7 8+		R = Yes

Scale	Cesarean section (prior)	Stillbirth/neonatal death (prior)	Thyroid problems	Toxemia (current)	Blood pressure problems	Weight
RROS						
OCS		R = Yes			R = >140/90	
HRPSS	R = Yes	R = Yes	R = Yes	R = Mild, moderate, or severe	R = Chronic hypertension	R = <100 lb >200 lb
MCHCI + LI	R = Yes	R = ⩾1 stillbirth ⩾1 neonatal	R = Yes	R = Mild or severe	R = Chronic: mild severe, or nephritis	R = Malnourished or very obese
UCNM		R = Neonatal		R = Yes		

Note. R = risk. Subjects failing to meet the risk criteria are assumed to be at no risk for that factor. From "Perinatal Outcome: The Similarity and Predictive Values of Antpartum and Intrapartum Assessment Scales" by V. J. Molfese, B. Thomson, and A. Bennett, 1985. *Journal of Reproductive Medicine, 30,* pp. 32–33. Copyright 1985 by the *Journal of Reproductive Medicine.* Reprinted by permission.

TABLE 3-6. Intrapartum Categories and Risk Definitions from Perinatal Risk Scales

Scale	Abnormal presentation	Amniotic fluid	Cord problems	Drugs in labor	Fetal heart rate	Forceps	Induced labor
RROS	R = Not vertex	R = Turbid or bloody	R = Knotted, prolapsed, tight, or nuchal	R = Analgesia > 50 mg; anesthesia > local or pudendal	R = Low	R = ≥ low	R = Yes
OCS	R = Not vertex	R = Not clear	R = Knotted, nuchal, or prolapsed	R = Yes	R = <100 beats/min >160 beats/min	R = > low	R = Yes
HRPSS	R = Breech or abnormal position	R = Meconium	R = Prolapsed	R = Specific types and doses	R = Bradycardia or tachycardia	R = Outlet or operative	R = Medical or elective
MCHCI + LI		R = Meconium			R = <115 beats/min >165 beats/min		
UCNM	R = Breech or abnormal position		R = Prolapsed				R = Yes or Pitocin stimulation

Scale	Length of labor	Multiple pregnancy	Premature rupture of membranes	Placenta problems	Cesarean section
RROS	R = Specific length/parity	R = Yes	R = Yes	R = Yes	R = Planned or unplanned
OCS	R = Specific length/stage	R = Yes	R = > 12 hr	R = Specific types	R = Yes
HRPSS	R = Specific length	R = Yes	R = > 12 hr	R = Specific types	R = Primary or repeat
MCHCI + LI		R = Yes	R = > 24 hr		
UCNM		R = Yes	R = Yes	R = Specific types	R = Yes

Note. R = risk. Subjects failing to meet the risk criteria are assumed to be at no risk for that factor. From "Perinatal Outcome: The Similarity and Predictive Values of Antepartum and Intrapartum Assessment Scales" by V. J. Molfese, B. Thomson, and A. Bennett, 1985. *Journal of Reproductive Medicine, 30,* pp. 34–35. Copyright 1985 by the *Journal of Reproductive Medicine.* Reprinted by permission.

compared with the antepartum subscales seem to reflect the greater similarity of the categories represented by the specific items contained on the scales. The item content of the intrapartum subscales appears to be more homogeneous than that of the antepartum subscales.

The items contained on the MCHCI + LI are particularly interesting to consider in a discussion of scale-item homogeneity. Although the MCHCI + LI, particularly its antepartum subscale, contains many items that are similar to those on the other scales, it includes some items that are unique. For example, this is the only scale that includes items pertaining to social, economic, and cultural information, which permits one to consider factors such as race, employment, income, and education. This scale also tends to include multiple items dealing with the different apsects of a complication. There are, for example, several items related to preterm bleeding, to generative tract disorders, and to specific problems encountered in prior infants. This specificity produces more in-depth coverage of these complications. However, such coverage is at the expense of item breadth—the MCHCI + LI addresses fewer different types of intrapartum complications than do the other scales.

The second cause of the differences in the magnitudes of correlations across scales and subscales may be the scales' use of different defining characteristics to assess risk. To determine what effects the different defining characteristics had on subjects' risk scores, 2 × 2 chi-square analyses were computed within each category where risk/no-risk matrices could be constructed for all possible nonredundant pairs of scales. For example, a risk/no-risk matrix was constructed for the UCNM and the HRPSS for the abortion category. This category was dichotomized according to whether risk points or no risk points were assigned to each subject on both scales. Such a matrix was also constructed for the UCNM and the OCS for the dichotomized abortion category. Similar matrices were constructed for the other pairs of scales and for the other categories that could be similarly dichotomized. The data used in each analysis were the number of subjects who fell into each of the four cells of the matrix.

The chi-square analyses revealed that the majority of the comparisons yielded no significant differences. Thus the assignment of risk points to specific perinatal conditions that characterized each subject was generally similar across scales. However, in 31% (or 27 of 88) of the possible risk/no-risk comparisons within the antepartum categories, there were significant ($p < .01$) differences. In contrast, 11% (or 8 of 71) of the possible risk/no-risk comparisons within the intrapartum categories were significantly different. Thus the defining characteristics used to assess risk points for the intrapartum items generally seem to be more homogeneous than those used for the antepartum items. This, too, might be responsible for the generally higher correlations found for the intrapartum subscales compared to those found for the antepartum subscales.

Predictive Values of the Antepartum and Intrapartum Risk Scores

Although the risk scores produced by the scales constitute an important aspect of scale evaluation, the most important aspect is scale validity as reflected by the predictive values of the scales. The predictive value of each of the five scales was assessed using stepwise multiple regression analyses. These analyses were executed in order to determine the extent to which the neonatal and maternal outcome measures could be predicted from scores on the antepartum and intrapartum subscales. In each analysis, items that were redundant with the outcome measures (e.g., items pertaining to birthweight and gestational age) or that were always associated with an outcome measure were deleted from the scales in order to avoid spuriously high correlations. For example, in analyses using cesarean section as an outcome measure, items that tend to be related to cesarean section procedures, such as administration of general anesthesia and previous cesarean section, were deleted from the scales.

Two sets of regression analyses were executed. The first set was executed in order to address the second research issue—the finding of Hobel *et al.* (1973) that intrapartum scores are more accurate than antepartum scores in predicting perinatal outcomes. Therefore, in this set of analyses, the intrapartum scores were entered into the equation first, followed by the antepartum scores. In the second set of analyses, antepartum scores were entered before intrapartum scores. In this way, it was possible to evaluate both the amount of change in the measurement variance that could be accounted for and the standardized beta weights that were produced by entering the intrapartum scores first versus that produced by entering the antepartum scores first. To verify the Hobel *et al.* finding, the amount of variance and the beta weights of the intrapartum scores had to be higher than those for the antepartum scores.

The results of both sets of stepwise multiple regression analyses, summarized in Table 3-7, were similar. The relative proportion of total variance explained by the antepartum scores versus that explained by the intrapartum scores did not differ when antepartum scores were entered into the equation before intrapartum scores or after. There were differences in the beta weights of the antepartum and intrapartum scores. The beta weights indicate the strength of the contribution of each type of score to the equation. In general, the beta weights of the antepartum scores were larger than those of the intrapartum scores for the neonatal outcome measures, but the intrapartum beta weights were larger for primary cesarean section. The beta weights were about equal for midforceps delivery.

The general pattern found in the results across scales is contrary to the assertion of Hobel *et al.* (1973) that "intrapartum events are in general more predictive [than antepartum events]" (p. 8). It should be kept in mind, however, that the specific outcome measure (days in the hospital) used by Hobel *et al.* in their regression analyses was not used in the study reported here. However, considering the results of equations using only the HRPSS scores, there is a predictive advantage for intrapartum over antepartum scores. Unfortunately, the regression models computed on the HRPSS were significant for only two of the outcome measures (neonatal subscale scores and incidence of primary cesarean section). With so few

Table 3-7. Results of Stepwise Multiple Regression Analyses

	Infant morbidity: Apgar 1-min	Infant morbidity: Apgar 5-min	Infant morbidity: GA	Infant morbidity: BWT	Infant morbidity: RDS	Infant morbidity: Neonatal subscale scores	Maternal morbidity: Primary CS
RROS			A .11 I .00 F = 6.90** R^2 = .11		A .14 I .01 F = 9.70** R^2 = .15	A .16 I .06 F = 14.77** R^2 = .22	A .03 I .28 F = 24.98** R^2 = .31
OCS					A .08 I .01 F = 5.40** R^2 = .09		A .12 I .07 F = 13.61** R^2 = .19
HRPSS						A .02 I .07 F = 4.86** R^2 = .09	A .00 I .41 F = 39.29** R^2 = .41
MCHCI + LI	A .05 I .03 F = 4.64** R^2 = .08	A .06 I .01 F = 4.50* R^2 = .07		A .00 I .08 F = 4.83** R^2 = .08	A .01 I .06 F = 3.95* R^2 = .07	A .05 I .08 F = 8.15** R^2 = .13	
UCNM	A .11 I .01 F = 7.87** R^2 = .12	A .10 I .02 F = 7.87** R^2 = .12	A .05 I .02 F = 4.53* R^2 = .07				A .01 I .20 F = 14.67** R^2 = .21

Note. Shown in the table are the F values with both antepartum (A) and intrapartum (I) scores entered in the equation; the R^2 values (the proportion of variance explained by the A and I predictors) for the A subscale and the I subscale; and the total R^2 values. GA = gestational age; BWT = birthweight; RDS = respiratory distress syndrome; CS = cesarean section. Adapted from "Perinatal Outcome: The Similarity and Predictive Values of Antepartum and Intrapartum Assessment Scales" by V. J. Molfese, B. Thomson, and A. Bennett, 1985. *Journal of Reproductive Medicine, 30,* p. 37. Copyright 1985 by the *Journal of Reproductive Medicine.* Adapted by permission.

*$p < .025$.

**$p < .01$.

significant results, it is difficult to assess the consistency of the Hobel *et al.* pattern.

From the various published arguments, it makes sense that intrapartum subscales should be better predictors than they were found to be across the scales in this study. The poorer predictive value of intrapartum scores might be due to the relatively small number of items on the intrapartum subscales compared to the number on the antepartum subscales. Most of the scales have a 60%–40% or 70%–30% antepartum to intrapartum split between the items they contain. If the split on the other scales more closely resembled that found on the HRPSS, perhaps the predictive value of the intrapartum scores could be improved.

Although none of the scales would predict all of the outcome measures shown in Table 3-7, each scale could predict some of these measures. The RROS could predict four of the eight outcome measures, with antepartum scores contributing more than intrapartum scores to the predictions of gestational age, respiratory distress, and neonatal subscale scores. Intrapartum scores contributed more only in predicting primary cesarean section. The OCS could predict respiratory distress and primary cesarean section, with antepartum scores contributing more to the prediction of both outcome measures. The HRPSS could predict neonatal subscale scores and the incidence of primary cesarean section. For both measures, intrapartum scores contributed more to the predictions. The most outcome measures—five of the eight—were predicted by the MCHCI + LI. There were no subscale differences in predicting 1-minute Apgar scores and neonatal subscale scores, but antepartum scores contributed more to predicting 5-minute Apgar scores, and intrapartum scores, to predicting birthweight and respiratory distress. The UCNM predicted four outcome measures. Intrapartum scores contributed more to the prediction of 1- and 5-minute Apgar scores and to the incidence of primary cesarean section. Antepartum scores were slightly stronger predictors of gestational age.

The scales were quite variable in their abilities to predict the infant outcome measures. The scale that best predicted these measures was the MCHCI + LI, which predicted all infant measures except gestational age. Interestingly, though the other scales produce similar risk scores (as determined by total and subscale correlations), they do not closely resemble each other in terms of the specific outcome measures that are predicted by the scores. Apparently these scales contain items and risk criteria that are different enough to produce different predictive values.

There was somewhat less variability across scales in the prediction of the maternal outcome measures. None of the scale scores could predict midforceps delivery, probably because of the low incidence of this outcome in the particular subject sample used for the study. Scores from all of the scales except the MCHCI + LI could predict the incidence of primary cesarean section. The highest predictive values, defined in terms of the proportion of the variance accounted for, were found for primary cesarean section. The specific intrapartum items included on the five scales seem particularly suitable for predicting this type of event.

Number of Complications versus Weighted Score as a Measure of Perinatal Risk

Because the scores assigned to all items on the perinatal risk scales are relatively arbitrary, except for those on the UCNM, which uses empirically determined risk weightings, it is still not known whether the items are appropriately weighted. Strobino and Baruffi (1984) reported that number of complications constituted a more valid and simpler measure of "risk" for the HRPSS neonatal subscale than did weighted scores. Prechtl (1967) also noted that number of complications is a useful indicator of risk. Indeed, both Prechtl's Optimal Obstetric Conditions Scale and the OCS (Littman & Parmelee) use number of complications as the basic risk score.

This issue of number of complications versus weighted score has never been examined for most of the perinatal risk scales and seems to be an appropriate comparison to make across scales. To address this third research issue, two sets of Pearson product–moment correlations were computed. In the first set, the usual weighted scores were used as the basis for the risk scores. In the second set, the scale items were weighted to reflect the number of complications only. These "unweighted" scores were then used as the basis for the risk scores. Because the items on the OCS were already unweighted (1 penalty point being awarded for each complication that is present), the correlations for the weighted scores and those for the unweighted scores for this scale were identical. The outcome measures used in both sets of analyses were birthweight, gestational age, 1- and 5-minute Apgar scores, and the neonatal items from the HRPSS.

The results of the two sets of correlational analyses are shown in Table 3-8 (Sample 1). As can be seen, the results were remarkably similar. Although the magnitudes of the correlations varied slightly, there were no cases in which significant correlations were produced between the weighted scale scores and the outcome measures but not between the unweighted scale scores and the outcome measures. It appears that there are no obvious advantages to using unweighted scores instead of weighted scores.

These findings were verified in a separate sample of 130 women and their infants. These women were participating in a prospective study involving the measurement of pregnancy attitudes and psychological traits during pregnancy and the measurement of perinatal risks, psychological traits, and infant status during the postpartum period. (Other information and descriptive statistics on this sample are contained in Chapter 6.) Pearson product–moment correlations were computed on data obtained from these women and their infants. Again, weighted and unweighted scores were used as perinatal risk scores. The correlations for both types of scores are shown in Table 3-8 (Sample 2). As can be seen, the weighted scores produced slightly higher correlations with the outcome measures than were produced by the number of complications. As a result, there were six instances in which there were significant correlations between weighted scores and particular outcome measures, and there was one instance in which there was a signifi-

TABLE 3-8. Results of Correlational Analyses Using Weighted and Unweighted Scale Scores

	Sample 1 (N = 116)					Sample 2 (N = 130)				
Scale	BWT	GA	1-min Apgar	5-min Apgar	HRPSS neonatal items	BWT	GA	1-min Apgar	5-min Apgar	HRPSS neonatal items
Correlations using number of complications										
RROS	−.21*	−.31**	−.30**	−.25**	.56**	.14	.22**	−.23**	−.20**	.18*
OCS	−.27**	−.33**	−.34**	−.24**	.52**	.01	.24**	−.14	−.17*	.17*
HRPSS	−.04	−.19*	−.30**	−.21*	.51**	.18*	.23**	−.18*	−.15*	.27**
MCHCI + LI	−.03	−.05	−.21*	−.31**	.05	.05	.09	−.08	−.09	.24**
UCNM	−.10	−.30**	−.24**	−.23**	.52**	.12	.16*	−.13	−.14	.12
Correlations using weighted scores										
RROS	−.16*	−.25**	−.28**	−.18*	.53**	.18*	.20**	−.23**	−.18*	.18*
OCS	−.27**	−.33**	−.34**	−.24**	.52**	.01	.24**	−.14	−.17*	.17*
HRPSS	−.06	−.19*	−.30**	−.18*	.54**	.15*	.24**	−.19*	−.21**	.28**
MCHCI + LI	−.10	−.17*	−.22**	−.20*	.26**	.06	.08	−.11	−.12	.30**
UCNM	.08	−.21**	−.48**	−.45**	.59**	.06	.14	−.15*	−.22**	.25**

Note. BWT = birthweight; GA = gestational age.

* $p < .05$.

** $p < .01$.

cant correlation between an unweighted score and a particular outcome measure. When considering the magnitudes of the correlations, there appears to be an advantage to using weighted scores instead of unweighted scores. However, the magnitude of the differences in correlation is small, ranging from .01 to .13.

It had been expected that the unweighted scores would prove to be better indicators of perinatal risk and, as such, more highly correlated with the outcome measures than the weighted scores. Analysis of the data from both samples of subjects does not support that expectation. Although the weighted scores assigned to the perinatal complications by scale developers have been criticized as being arbitrary, the weightings do not appear to be inappropriate.

SUMMARY

The results of these analyses provide considerable information on how the five perinatal risk scales compare in terms of the scores they generate for individual subjects and how useful the scores are for predicting specific outcome measures. Four of the five scales produced fairly similar total scale scores. However, the overall predictive values of these scores were not as good as the predictive value of the scores derived from the least similar scale. The major differences among the scales seem to lie in the specific antepartum items they contain rather than in the intrapartum items. In general, the intrapartum items are quite similar.

The results also show that scores from the scales can be used, with varying degrees of success, to predict neonatal and maternal outcome measures. Although some scales enable one to predict a variety of outcome measures from their scores, it might be possible to improve the predictions by adding new items or by reformulating the scales. This issue of constructing a new, composite scale is explored in Chapter 5.

Finally, it appears that there is an advantage to using weighted scores rather than number of complications (unweighted scores) as a measure of perinatal risk. Higher correlation coefficients were obtained when weighted risk scores were used, contrary to the predictions of Strobino and Baruffi (1980) and Prechtl (1967). Although risk weightings are, for the most part, arbitrarily assigned to perinatal risk items, the scores do seem to be significantly related to the outcome measures.

CHAPTER

4

Complications versus Optimality: Theoretical Bases of Perinatal Risk Scales

The purpose of perinatal risk assessment scales is to screen women during pregnancy and/or labor for factors that place them at risk for negative outcomes. Once screened, the women identified as being at risk can be referred for specific follow-up care or treatment. Two different approaches have been taken with regard to what the focal point should be during the perinatal period. One approach focuses on the abnormal conditions in pregnancy and labor that produce negative outcomes. These abnormal conditions are seen as the targets to be identified during perinatal screening. This approach has resulted in the development of what are commonly referred to as "complication scales," or scales that contain items with defining characteristics that identify the "abnormal" region, that is, the region that lies outside the normal range. For example, perinatal complications arise more often in women who are under 18 years of age or over 35. Risk points are thus assigned to such women but not to women who fall within the "normal" range, between the ages of 18 and 35 years. The goal of these types of scales is to adjust the risk score values so that the sensitivity rate is low enough to detect the abnormal cases without identifying a large percentage of cases that are not abnormal.

The second approach focuses on the conditions in pregnancy and labor that are most likely to produce positive outcomes. This approach is associated with what are commonly called "optimality scales." Prechtl (1981) has argued that the optimality approach is more accurate than complication scales in predicting normal outcomes because it uses narrower criteria to define optimality than those used on complication scales. Thus only mothers with perinatal characteristics that fall within the normal range would be considered as having "optimal" status, and their infants would more likely be optimal as well. Prechtl (1967) noted that a simple count of the number of nonoptimal items could be used as a means of identifying women who are or are not at risk for poor perinatal outcomes, since more than one nonoptimal item places a woman at risk.

There are additional, functional differences in the approaches associated with the use of complication scales versus the use of optimality scales. Researchers who use complication scales tend to view them as a basis for selecting subjects for study or intervention. Those who use complication scales also seem to be more interested in using them for the purpose of describing their research subjects in terms of the level of medical risk (e.g., high, medium, and low). The tendency to use these scales for grouping subjects is reflected in the fact that risk score categories are usually provided by the scales.

Optimality scales, on the other hand, at least the early ones, have been used more as a means of predicting perinatal outcomes than as a means of categorizing subjects. Prechtl's (1967) original use of optimality scores (Scale of Optimal Obstetric Conditions; OOC) was to predict neurological functioning at birth, because such functioning had been found to be predictive of later development. Prechtl later used risk categories to predict neurological status in infancy. Most frequently, however, optimal scores tend to be used as continuous rather than categorical variables. Littman and Parmelee's (1978) Obstetrical Complication's Scale (OCS) is another optimality scale that utilizes continuous rather than categorical scores. Indeed, the OCS provides a conversion scale by which continuous scale scores can be converted to continuous standard scores. These differences in approach to scale use have resulted in some differences in the types of screening efforts to which these scales have been applied.

Several issues have arisen in the literature concerning the predictive superiority of complication scales over optimality scales. These issues have not been resolved on the basis of empirical evidence. Indeed, comparisons of the results of studies using optimality scales with those of studies using complication scales to predict various neonatal and infant outcome measures do not show a clear advantage of one type of scale over the other in terms of magnitude of correlations, accuracy of classifications, or predicted outcomes. Such comparisons, however, are of questionable validity because of the wide differences across studies in the populations sampled, the statistical procedures used, and the outcome variables measured. The issue of which type of scale is able to predict perinatal outcome measures more accurately needs to be addressed under more controlled conditions. There are, however, differences between the optimality-based scales and the complication-based scales that make direct comparisons difficult. These differences are described in the sections that follow.

DIFFERENCES BETWEEN COMPLICATION AND OPTIMALITY SCALES

Differences in Risk Scoring

In developing the optimality concept, Prechtl (1968) and Littman and Parmelee (1978) devised scales with characteristics that they believed were quite different from those of traditional complication scales. The scales developed by both Prechtl and Littman and Parmelee use a weighting system whereby the presence of each complication, or nonoptimal condition, receives a 1-point penalty and all conditions are weighted the same. Because only 1-point penalties are assessed, many nonoptimal conditions must be present before a major deviation from optimality is reflected in the scores. Prechtl (1967, 1968) and others (Parmelee, Kopp, & Sigman, 1976) have discussed the use of this weighting system, noting that nonoptimal conditions do not usually occur in isolation. Thus the presence of one nonoptimal condition is likely to give rise to another nonoptimal condition, and these, in turn, give rise to a chain of nonoptimal conditions. The result is a high nonoptimal score.

In a recent study by Rosenberg *et al.* (1981), 314,153 birth certificates were examined in order to obtain information on the issue of the cumulative nature of complications. The reseachers analyzed the data to determine if the number of intrapartum complications was higher for women who had had one or more antepartum complications. Cases were divided into four groups: those with a previous fetal loss, those with antepartum complications or diseases, those with both prior fetal loss and antepartum complications or diseases, and those with no complications. There were significantly more intrapartum complications in cases with antepartum complications/diseases and in cases with both fetal loss and antepartum complications/diseases. These findings can be interpreted as providing support for the assertion that complications tend not to occur in isolation but are cumulative. The cumulative nature of perinatal complications was also revealed in Strobino and Baruffi's (1984) study of the validity of the neonatal items on the Hobel *et al.* scale (the High-Risk Pregnancy Screening System; HRPSS). The complication items were found to cluster together more often than they were found to exist in isolation.

The cumulative nature of complications is also acknowledged in complication-based scales (e.g., Goodwin *et al.,* 1969; Hobel *et al.,* 1973; Morrison & Olsen, 1979). However, instead of using an equal weighting system, these scales typically assign heavier weights to conditions that are thought to be of serious consequence to infant outcome. Lesser weights are assigned to conditions that are thought to be of less serious consequence. With this sytem, women with more serious complications will have larger total risk scores than women with less serious complications. This would generally be true even if there were a greater number of the less serious complications because of the magnitude of the scores used.

The weightings assigned to specific antepartum, intrapartum, and postpartum items on the optimality and complications scales are shown in Tables 4-1, 4-2, and 4-3, respectively. Perinatal conditions that were present on two or more of these scales were included as categories in the tables. There are 23 antepartum items, 13 intrapartum items, and 6 postpartum

TABLE 4-1. Antepartum Scale Items and Risk Definitions

Scale	Abortion	Age	Albuminuria	Anemia	Birthweight of prior infants	Bleeding	Drugs in pregnancy
UCNM		r = <17 yr >30 yr			r = Low		
RROS	r = >2	r = <16 yr primigravida <18 yr multigravida >35 yr					r = Chronic medication
HRPSS	$\underline{r}$ = Habitual abortion	$\underline{r}$ = ≤15 yr >35 yr		r = <9–10.9 gm Hb	$\underline{r}$ = >10 lb	$\underline{r}$ = Spotting	r = Smoke ≥ 1 pack/day, alcohol (moderate use)
OOC	r = > 2	r = <18 yr primigravida <20 yr multigravida >30 yr	r = With edema	r = <7 hematocrit		r = Yes	
OCS	r = > 2	r = <18 yr >30 yr	r = Yes	r = <10 gm Hb		r = Yes	r = Yes

Scale	Chronic or acute disorders/diseases	Fertility problems	Gyn. problems	Hyperemesis	Parity	Pelvis	Prenatal care
UCNM	R = Specific disease		R = Specific problems				r = 0 visits 1–3 4–7 8+
RROS	r–R = Chronic diseases or infections present				r = >6		
HRPSS	r–R = Chronic and specific acute disorders/ diseases present		r–R = Specific problems		r = >5		
OOC	r = Chronic and specific acute disorders/ diseases present	r = Unwanted sterility >2 yr		r = Yes	r = 0 >6	r = Disproportion	
OCS	r = Chronic and specific acute disorders/ diseases present	r = Unwanted sterility		r = Yes	r = 0 >6	r = Disproportion	r = Not in 1st half of pregnancy

(continued)

TABLE 4-1. *(Continued)*

Scale	Premature infant (prior)	Rh problems (prior)	Stillbirth/ neonatal death (prior)	Stress/ emotion	Surgery/ X-ray (abdominal)	Toxemia (current)	Blood pressure problems	Marital status	Weight or nutrition
UCNM		R = Yes	r = Neonatal		r̲ = Yes	r̲ = Yes			
RROS									
HRPSS	R = Yes	r–R = Sensitization	R = Yes	r = Emotional problems		r̲–R = Mild, moderate, or severe	r = Chronic hypertension		r̲ = <100 >200
OOS		r = Antagonism or incompatibility		r = Stress	r = X-ray	r = > Mild	r = >90/135	r = Unmarried	r = Not well nourished
OCS	r = Yes	r = Antagonism or incompatibility	r = Stillbirth				r = >140/90	r = Not married	

Note. r = low risk; r̲ = medium risk; R = high risk. Subjects failing to meet the risk criteria are assumed to be at no risk for that factor. From "Optimality versus Complications: Assessing Predictive Values of Perinatal Scales" by V. J. Molfese and B. K. Thomson, 1985. *Child Development, 56,* pp. 814–815.

infant items that have been derived from the five perinatal risk scales. Three of the five scales are complication scales (the UCNM, the HRPSS, and the RROS) and two are optimality scales (the OOC and the OCS). To simplify the tables, symbols were used to indicate risk points. The exact risk probabilities utilized by the Brazie *et al.* scale (cited in Lubchenco, 1976) (UCNM) as risk points have been grouped and coded as r = <10 points, r̲ = 10–20 points, and R = > 20 points. The codes for the other scales are as follows: Zax *et al.* scale (1977) (RROS)—r = 1 point, r̲ = 2 points, and R = 3–4 points; Hobel *et al.* scale (1973) (HRPSS)—r = 1 point, r̲ = 5 points, R = 10 points. For purposes of comparison, the optimality scales of Prechtl (1967) (OOC) and Littman and Parmelee (1978) (OCS) are also shown in the tables. For these latter scales, r = 1 point.

The differences in the weighting systems used by the scales can be seen in the tables. Because of the differences in the magnitude of the item scores, we would expect there to be greater differences in scores among subjects on complication scales than on optimality scales. Differences in the variability of the scores generated by complication versus optimality scales for each subject might be sufficient to affect the overall predictive values of the scales.

The weighting systems used by optimality scales and complication scales lend themselves to an examination of the issue, described in Chapter 3, of whether number of complications or risk score is a more accurate predictor of perinatal outcome. Optimality scale scores are calculated simply by tallying the number of complications that are present. Since all items on optimality scales have the same weight, the optimality score reflects a measure of number of complications. On complication scales, however, each complication has a weighted score assigned to it. Thus the complication scale score reflects the number of complications plus a multiplier reflecting the presumed impact of each complication on perinatal outcome. If, as Strobino and Baruffi (1984) and Prechtl (1967) have claimed, number of complications is a more accurate predictor than weighted score, optimality scales should show an advantage over complication scales. As reported in Chapter 3, however, the weighted scores examined in the Molfese *et al.* (1985) study

TABLE 4-2. Intrapartum Scale Items and Risk Definitions

Scale	Abnormal presentation	Amniotic fluid	Cord problems	Drugs in labor	Fetal heart rate	Forceps	Induced labor
UCNM	$\underline{r}$ = Breech or abnormal position		$\underline{r}$ = Prolapsed				R = Yes or Pitocin stimulation
RROS	r = Not vertex	r–$\underline{r}$ = Turbid or bloody	r = Knotted, prolapsed, or tight	r–$\underline{r}$ = Analgesia > 50 mg; anesthesia > local or pudenal	$\underline{r}$ = Low	r–$\underline{r}$ = ⩾ Low	r = Yes
HRPSS	R = Breech or abnormal position	$\underline{r}$–R = Meconium	R = Prolapsed	$\underline{r}$ = Specific types and doses	R = Bradycardia or tachycardia	r–$\underline{r}$ = Outlet or vacuum	R–$\underline{r}$ = Medical or elective
OOC	r = Not vertex	r = Not clear	r = Nuchal, prolapsed, or knotted	r = >O_2 and local	r = < 100 beats/min >160 beats/min Not regular		
OCS	r = Not vertex	r = Not clear	r = Knotted, nuchal, or prolapsed	r = Yes	r = < 100 beats/min >160 beats/min	r = > Low	r = Yes

Scale	Length of labor	Multiple pregnancy	Premature rupture of membranes	Placenta problems	Cesarean section	Spontaneous delivery
UCNM		r = Yes	$\underline{r}$ = Yes	R = Specific types	r = Yes	
RROS	r–$\underline{r}$ = Long or short	r = Yes	r = Yes	r = Yes	r–$\underline{r}$ = Planned or unplanned	
HRPSS	r–$\underline{r}$ = Specific length	R = Yes	$\underline{r}$ = > 12 hr	r–R = Specific types	$\underline{r}$ = Primary or repeat	
OOC	r = Specific length/stage	r = Yes	r = < 6 hr	r = Specific types		r = No
OCS	r = Specific length/stage	r = Yes	r = > 12 hr	r = Specific types		r = No

Note. r = low risk; $\underline{r}$ = medium risk; R = high risk. Subjects failing to meet the risk criteria are assumed to be at no risk for that factor. From "Optimality versus Complications: Assessing Predictive Values of Perinatal Scales" by V. J. Molfese and B. K. Thomson, 1985. *Child Development, 56,* pp. 815–816. Copyright 1985 by the Society for Research in Child Development, Inc. Reprinted by permission.

TABLE 4-3. Postpartum Scale Items and Risk Definitions

Scale	Apgar	Birthweight	Disorders/ anomalies	Gestational age	Respiration onset	Resuscitation treatment
UCNM						r = Active
RROS	r = <8 at 5 min	r = < 2,500 gm and/or premature	r̲ = Physical or gross anomaly			r = Yes
HRPSS	r̲–R = <5 at 5 min <5 at 1 min	r̲–R = < 2,000 or 2,000–2,500 gm	r–R = Anomalies or specific disorders	r̲–R = Dysmaturity Prematurity > 42 wk		R = Yes
OOC		r = < 2,000 gm > 4,900 gm	r = Specific disorders	r = < 38 wk >41 wk	r = > 1 min	r = Yes
OCS	r–R = <7 at 1 min <7 at 5 min	r = < 2,500 gm		r = < 37 wk	r = > 6 min	r = Yes

Note. r = low risk; r̲ = medium risk; R = high risk. Subjects failing to meet the risk criteria are assumed to be at no risk for that factor. From "Optimality versus Complications: Assessing Predictive Values of Perinatal Scales" by V. J. Molfese and B. K. Thomson, 1985. *Child Development, 56,* p. 816. Copyright 1985 by the Society for Research in Child Development, Inc. Reprinted by permission.

tended to have higher correlations with outcome measures than did the unweighted scores. This issue of the relationship of weighted versus unweighted scores to outcome measures was addressed in a reanalysis of data obtained in another study, conducted by Molfese and Thomson (1985) and described later in this chapter. Both optimality scales are contrasted with the three complication scales in the reanalysis.

Differences in Scale Items and Definitions

The optimality and complication scales appear to contain similar items with similar defining characteristics. In an effort to compare items contained on these scales, the items on two optimality scales (the OCS and the OOC) and three complication scales (the UCNM, the HRPSS, and the RROS) were categorized as shown in Tables 4-1, 4-2, and 4-3. The majority of items on the scales fit into common categories. Each scale did contain some unique items, but the percentage of such items was small, ranging from 7% to 11%. The major differences among the scales lie in the number of items they contain and the defining characteristics they use to identify the risk conditions. The number of items on the scales ranges from 25 to 126. Interestingly, the scales with the most items do not necessarily cover more risk conditions. Rather, these longer scales tend to cover more specific aspects of certain conditions than are covered by the other scales. For example, all the scales include an item pertaining to chronic and acute diseases, but some scales incorporate a variety of conditions pertaining to specific chronic and acute diseases rather than using just a single, comprehensive item.

The characteristics defining the range of risk for each item on the five scales are also shown in Tables 4-1, 4-2, and 4-3. In general, the scales use similar defining characteristics for their risk conditions, although the optimality scales, compared to the complication scales, tend to use definitions with a narrower range of variability for some items. For example, on optimality scales, the range of risk for maternal age is under 18 years and over 30 years; on complication scales, this range is under 15 or

18 years and over 35 years. These differences in the definitions applied to the scale items should produce differences in the perinatal risk scores obtained by an individual on the various scales, that is, an individual may be considered to be "at risk" on the basis of optimality scale scores but not on the basis of complication scale scores.

Differences in Validation Studies

There are also differences between optimality scales and complication scales in the types of studies that have been used to validate them. Optimality scales have often been validated by studies using outcome measures that were selected because of their behavioral relevance (e.g., neurological assessment, postnatal complications, Brazelton Neonatal Behavioral Assessment Scale scores, Gesell scale scores, and Bayley scale scores). Complication scales have most often been validated by studies using medically relevant outcome measures (e.g., mortality rates, incidence of meconium, cesarean section rates, and days in intensive care). Although these two types of outcome measures are not mutually exclusive, there do tend to be differences in the types of outcome measures that are used in the studies conducted to validate each type of scale. Because of these differences, it is difficult to compare the validity of perinatal risk scores across both types of scales.

Retrospective versus Prospective Studies

Optimality and complication scales have been used in studies that often differ in terms of research design. Optimality scales have been used most frequently in studies with retrospective designs—those in which a target population is identified (e.g., low birthweight infants, infants of teenaged mothers) and medical histories (i.e., antepartum, intrapartum, and postpartum histories) of subjects are examined for the critical variables to be studied. Complications scales, however, have most frequently been used in prospective research or for prospective applications. In prospective designs, a target population is identified (e.g., pregnant teenagers) and measurements of the critical variables are obtained throughout the study period (i.e., the antepartum, intrapartum, and/or postpartum periods).

The retrospective and prospective research designs can, in perinatal research, produce quite different results because of differences in the types of studies than can be done. For example, the retrospective design may preclude the assessment of some outcomes (e.g., perinatal mortality) if a specific target population (e.g., women whose pregnancies resulted in live births) is selected as the subject sample. In addition, because retrospective data are collected after some particular target event or period has occurred (e.g., the postpartum period), the measures that can be examined relevant to conditions that existed prior to the target event are limited by what information happens to be available. Prospective designs also influence the types of studies that can be done. Studies that utilize prospective designs cover longer periods of time than those using retrospective designs because of the time lapse between the occurrence of the target event (e.g., an initial prenatal visit) and the time at which the final measures are obtained (e.g., postpartum outcome measures). Because studies of this type are more time consuming, they tend to be more expensive. Prospective designs, however, have an advantage over retrospective designs because they rely less on historical records for data and thus are less restricted in terms of the conditions they are able to examine. Data in prospective studies can be collected according to the specifications of the study throughout the study period.

Both retrospective and prospective designs are vulnerable to problems of sampling bias. Some types of subjects are more likely to be sampled than other types by these designs because of testing-site preferences. For example, in studies using retrospective designs, postpartum patients are the most frequently studied group of subjects because of their accessibility. Some types of postpartum patients are more available for testing than others, such as cesarean section patients, who are hospitalized longer than patients who have delivered vaginally. Because the cesarean section patient has different perinatal characteristics than the patient who has delivered vaginally, the data obtained from the former can be biased. In prospective designs, women receiving prenatal care are more often used as subjects because they can be easily accessed in early pregnancy in large numbers through clinics and prenatal classes. However, patients with specific types of perinatal risks or subject characteristics may be selectively served by the clinics and prenatal classes compared to women who do not seek such services early in pregnancy. As a result, there can be a sampling bias. In addition, because of the longer study period involved in prospective designs, these studies are vulnerable to potential bias resulting from subject attrition. Differences between subjects who complete their participation in a study and those who drop out prior to completion may affect the data, so that the results are invalid or unreliable.

Since the use of one design over the other is not dictated by the characteristics of either the optimality or the complication scales, it is possible to use either retrospective or prospective research designs for studying both types of perinatal risk scales. However, the performance of optimality and complication scales in both types of research designs has not been systematically studied. It is reasonable to expect that the type of research design used will have an effect on the type of results obtained with the scales, since the subjects sampled under each design are likely to have different characteristics.

Differences in Reproductive Phases Evaluated

Differences also exist between optimality and complication scales in terms of what reproductive phases they evaluate. The two optimality scales reviewed here (the OOC and the OCS) include items covering the antepartum, intrapartum, and postpartum periods. However, this is not generally true of traditional complication scales. Some complication scales evaluate only the antepartum period (e.g., Goodwin *et al.,* 1969; Nesbitt & Aubry, 1969), some only the intrapartum period (e.g., Morrison *et al.,* 1980), and others both the antepartum and intrapartum periods (e.g., Nesbitt & Aubry, 1969; Aubry & Pennington, 1973). All three periods are evaluated on only a few of the complication scales, three of which are the UCNM, the HRPSS, and the RROS. Since all three reproductive phases are included on these latter complication scales, they are good scales to use in comparisons with optimality scales.

COMPARING PREDICTIVE VALIDITY: A RETROSPECTIVE STUDY

Taken together, the difference between optimality and complication scales make direct comparisons of their predictive validity problematical. However, three complication scales—the UCNM, the HRPSS, and the RROS—were found to be similar to optimality scales in that they use a cumulative scoring system, have been validated on behaviorally relevant outcome measures, and have items pertaining to the antepartum, intrapartum, and postpartum periods. These scales were used, along with two optimality scales—the OCS and the OOC—in a retrospective study by Molfese and Thomson (1985) that was designed to determine whether optimality scales are superior to complication scales in predicting neonatal and infant outcome measures.

Description of the Study

The study sample consisted of 103 women and their infants. These women volunteered to participate in the research and agreed to have their medical records and those of their infants evaluated for perinatal risks. The women also agreed to allow their infants to be assessed at birth on the Brazelton Neonatal Behavioral Assessment Scale and the Postnatal Complications Scale (PNCS) (see Table 2-6) and to be evaluated at 6 months of age on the Bayley Scales of Infant Development, the revised Carey Infant Temperament Questionnaire, and the Pediatric Complications Scale—4 Months (PCS) (see Table 2-7). The women ranged in age from 15 to 38 years ($\bar{x}$ = 26.03 years). All of them delivered live infants, 25 by cesarean section, of which 16 were primary and 9 were repeat sections. The infants' birthweights ranged from 2,353 to 5,215 grams ($\bar{x}$ = 3,472.4 grams); gestational ages, from 34 to 44 weeks ($\bar{x}$ = 39.7 weeks); and 1-minute and 5-minute Apgar scores, from 3 to 9 ($\bar{x}$ = 7.8) and from 7 to 10 ($\bar{x}$ = 8.9), respectively.

Of the 103 women who participated during the immediate postpartum period, 77 were available for the 6-month retesting. The unavailable women had moved, could not be reached by letter or phone, or were not interested in participating. Compared to the women who were available for testing, the unavailable women did not differ significantly on any of the perinatal variables being studied.

The five perinatal risk scales were scored during the postpartum period on the basis of information that was obtained from medical records. Data relevant to the antepartum period were taken from antepartum medical records, intrapartum data were taken from labor and delivery records, and postpartum data from postpartum and nursery records of the neonates' status until discharge. In each case, the scores were determined by using the exact parameters specified on each scale. Scores on each scale represent the number of actual risk points accumulated by each subject.

Descriptive statistics on the five scales are as follows: the UCNM—mean = 22.03, *SD* = 20.28, range = 2.2 to 152.4; the HRPSS—mean = 11.7, *SD* = 14.6, range = 0 to 70; the OCS—mean = 3.9, *SD* = 2.39, range = 0 to 13; the OOC—mean = 1.96, *SD* = 2.16, range = 0 to 10; the RROS—mean = 2.40, *SD* = 2.28, range = 0 to 10.

The outcome measures used to evaluate the predictive validity of the perinatal scales included commonly used measures as well as the postpartum status items contained on each scale. The neonatal outcome measures were birthweight, gestational age, 1- and 5-minute Apgar scores, the four subscales and the total scale of the Brazelton Neonatal Behavioral Assessment Scale (Als, 1978; Brazelton, 1973), the PNCS (Littman & Parmelee, 1978), and each scale's own group of neonatal status items (i.e., the neonatal status subscale). In analyses involving the latter measure, only the antepartum and intrapartum subscales were used as the scale scores. The outcome measures used to evaluate the infants at age 6 months were the

PCS—9 Months (Littman & Parmelee, 1978) (see Table 2-7), mental scores (MDI) from the Bayley Scales of Infant Development (Bayley, 1969), and the revised Carey Infant Temperament Questionnaire (Carey & McDevitt, 1978). Scores on the neonatal and infant scales used as outcome measures are shown in Table 4-4.

The data were analyzed in several ways in order to answer questions concerning the similarity of risk scores across scales and the validity of these scores for predicting neonatal and infant outcome measures. Pearson product–moment correlations were computed so as to determine the relationship between subjects' risk scores across scales. As can be seen in Table

TABLE 4-4. Scores on Neonatal and Infant Outcome Measures

Outcome measure	Mean	*SD*	Range
Brazelton Neonatal Behavioral Assessment Scale			
Interactive Processes	2.67	1.44	1–5
Motoric Processes	2.42	.89	1–5
Organization/State	2.13	1.07	1–5
Organization/Stress	2.12	1.28	1–5
Total scale	9.3	3.10	4–16
PNCS	1.02	.88	0–4
Neonatal status subscale			
UNCM	7.83	4.23	0–36.3
RROS	.24	.62	0–3
HRPSS	2.62	5.92	0–35
OOC	.22	.98	0–9
OCS	.20	.57	0–4
PCS—9 months	.99	1.28	0–9
Bayley Scales of Infant Development			
Mental Scale	117.96	14.68	66–144
Carey Infant Temperament Questionnaire			
Activity	4.22	.63	2.9–5.5
Rhythmicity	2.45	.80	1–4.42
Approach/Withdrawal	2.34	.76	1–4
Adaptability	2.25	.55	1–3.27
Intensity	3.34	.65	1.56–4.6
Mood	2.82	.67	1.5–4.7
Persistence	3.20	.76	1.63–5.29
Distractibility	2.22	.59	1–3.4
Threshold	3.94	.74	2.43–5.38

Note. From "Optimality versus Complications: Assessing Predictive Values of Perinatal Scales" by V. J. Molfese and B. K. Thomson, 1985. *Child Development, 56,* p. 812. Copyright 1985 by the Society for Research in Child Development, Inc. Reprinted by permission.

4-5, correlations for total scale scores range from .43 to .80, with the higher correlations occurring between the RROS, the HRPSS, the OOC, and the OCS. Separate correlations for the antepartum, intrapartum, and postpartum subscales are shown in Table 4-6. The antepartum subscale correlations range from .07 to .77, and the intrapartum correlations, from .46 to .94. The highest correlations on both subscales are between the two optimality scales (the OOC and the OCS). The postpartum subscale correlations range from .22 to .63, with the highest correlations occurring between the OCS and the UCNM, RROS, and HRPSS scales, respectively.

The scales' power to predict the outcome measures was examined using multiple regression. For the neonatal outcome measures, the *F* values in each analysis were derived from equations in which the antepartum subscale scores were entered first, followed by the intrapartum subscale scores. For the infant outcome measures, variables were entered into the equations following the same antepartum, intrapartum sequence, followed by the entry of the postpartum scores. The *F* and *R* values for those outcome measures that could be predicted are shown in Table 4-7. Because the Brazelton Interactive Processes, Organization/State, and Organization/Stress subscale scores and the PC Scale Scores could not be predicted from any scale, these measures are not included in the table. Also shown in Table 4-7 are the Pearson product–moment correlations (r) between outcome measures and total scale scores. Interestingly, the simple correlations are nearly identical to the multiple correlations produced in the multiple regression analyses by entering the subscales in separate steps.

TABLE 4-5. Correlation Coefficients for Total Scale Scores

Scale	UCNM	RROS	HRPSS	OOC	OCS
UCNM	×				
RROS	.51	×			
HRPSS	.57	.73	×		
OOC	.53	.65	.62	×	
OCS	.43	.73	.62	.80	×

Note. All correlations > .23 are significant ($p < .01$). From "Optimality versus Complications: Assessing Predictive Values of Perinatal Scales" by V. J. Molfese and B. K. Thomson, 1985. *Child Development, 56*, p. 818. Copyright 1985 by the Society for Research in Child Development, Inc. Reprinted by permission.

TABLE 4-6. Correlation Coefficients for Subscale Scores

Scale	Antepartum subscale					Intrapartum subscale					Postpartum subscale				
	UCNM	RROS	HRPSS	OOC	OCS	UCNM	RROS	HRPSS	OOC	OCS	UCNM	RROS	HRPSS	OOC	OCS
UCNM	×					×					×				
RROS	.07	×				.53	×				.32	×			
HRPSS	.18	.32	×			.55	.82	×			.34	.30	×		
OOC	.35	.27	.39	×		.61	.68	.60	×		.35	.22	.24	×	
OCS	.21	.43	.50	.77	×	.46	.66	.59	.94	×	.63	.56	.54	.31	×

Note. All correlations > .23 are significant ($p < .01$). From "Optimality versus Complications: Assessing Predictive Values of Perinatal Scales" by V. J. Molfese and B. K. Thomson, 1985. *Child Development, 56*, p. 818. Copyright 1985 by the Society for Research in Child Development, Inc. Reprinted by permission.

TABLE 4-7. Outcome Measures Predicted by Multiple Regression Analyses

Scale	Gestational age	1-minute Apgar	5-minute Apgar	Brazelton scale scores: Motoric Processes	Brazelton scale scores: Total	PNCS
UCNM			F = 6.72** R = .34 r = −.33**	F = 3.21 R = .25 r = −.25**		F = 3.87* R = .31 r = .32**
HRPSS		F = 4.25** R = .28 r = −.13	F = 8.91** R = .39 r = −.15			
RROS	F = 4.11* R = .26 r = −.08			F = 3.29* R = .30 r = −.08	F = 2.77* R = .28 r = −.12	F = 3.43* R = .28 r = .28**
OOC						
OCS						

Scale	Neonatal status	Bayley—Mental	Carey Infant Temperament Questionnaire: Activity	Carey Infant Temperament Questionnaire: Intensity	Carey Infant Temperament Questionnaire: Distractibility	Primary cesarean section
UCNM		$F = 2.77^*$	$F = 3.00^*$	$F = 3.09^*$		$F = 19.29^{**}$
		$R = .33$	$R = .36$	$R = .36$		$R = .53$
		$r = .31^{**}$	$r = .30^{**}$	$r = .32^{**}$		$r = .56^{**}$
HRPSS				$F = 4.56^{**}$		$F = 15.78^{**}$
				$R = .33$		$R = .49$
				$r = .36^{**}$		$r = .55^{**}$
RROS	$F = 3.44^*$			$F = 6.22^{**}$		$F = 5.84^{**}$
	$R = .28$			$R = .42$		$R = .31$
	$r = .07$			$r = .42^{**}$		$r = .58^{**}$
OOC	$F = 3.97^*$			$F = 5.17^{**}$	$F = 3.00^*$	$F = 16.77^{**}$
	$R = .26$			$R = .44$	$R = .36$	$R = .50$
	$r = .07$			$r = .42^{**}$	$r = .33^{**}$	$r = .50^{**}$
OCS				$F = 7.49^{**}$		$F = 6.75^{**}$
				$R = .44$		$R = .34$
				$r = .45^{**}$		$r = .40^{**}$

Note. From "Optimality versus Complications: Assessing Predictive Values of Perinatal Scales" by V. J. Molfese and B. K. Thomson, 1985. *Child Development, 56*, p. 819. Copyright 1985 by the Society for Research in Child Development, Inc. Reprinted by permission.
$^*p < .05$.
$^{**}p < .01$.

To directly compare the contribution of optimality scales versus that of complication scales in predicting outcomes, two additional multiple regression analyses were computed for each of the neonatal, infant, and maternal outcome measures. In the first analysis, scores from the two optimality scales (the OCS and the OOC) were entered first, followed by scores from the three complication scales (the UCNM, the HRPSS, and the RROS). In the second analysis, the complication scale scores were entered first, followed by the optimality scale scores. For 20 of the 27 outcome measures, the complication scale scores contributed more to the total R^2 value than did the optimality scale scores.

The issue of number of complications versus weighted scores as a measure of perinatal risk was also addressed in this study, as it was in the study discussed in Chapter 3. Table 4-8 shows the Pearson product–moment correlations for each of the five perinatal risk scales. In one set of correlations, weighted scores that were proposed by the scales' developers were used as risk scores. In the second set, unweighted scores

TABLE 4-8. Results of Correlational Analyses Using Weighted and Unweighted Scores

Scale	Birthweight	Gestational age	1-min Apgar	5-min Apgar	HRPSS neonatal items
		Correlations using weighted scores			
UCNM	.20*	−.005	−.11	−.32**	.25**
HRPSS	−.18*	−.10	−.22*	−.16	.57**
RROS	−.07	−.08	−.22*	−.22*	.27**
OCS	−.04	−.19*	−.23**	−.19*	.21*
OOC	−.03	−.15	−.15	−.16	.23*
		Correlations using number of complications			
UCNM	−.16	−.06	−.01	−.08	.29**
HRPSS	−.22*	−.04	−.15	−.02	.44**
RROS	−.03	−.12	−.23**	−.23**	.27**
OCS	−.04	−.19*	−.23**	−.19*	.21*
OOC	−.03	−.15	−.15	−.16	.23*

*$p < .05$.
**$p < .01$.

corresponding to a count of the total number of complications were used as risk scores. In general, the results show that there is some advantage to the weighted scores over the unweighted scores both in the magnitudes of the correlations and in the number of significant results. These results, obtained with yet a third subject sample, are consistent with those reported in Chapter 3.

Discussion of Study Results

The comparisons of scores generated by optimality scales with those generated by complication scales produced some interesting findings. The results of the correlational analyses revealed similarities as well as differences among the five scales. The total scale and the antepartum and intrapartum subscales of the OOC and the OCS (the two optimality scales) are highly similar. Much lower are the total scale and the antepartum and intrapartum subscale correlations among the UCNM, the HRPSS, and the RROS (the three complication scales). The postpartum subscales on the two optimality scales are not highly related, but the OCS postpartum subscale is highly related to the postpartum subscales of the three complication scales.

That similarities were found to exist between the two optimality scales is not surprising, given that the OCS contains items derived from the OOC and that the two scales utilize the same scoring system. The lack of similarity between the postpartum subscales may reflect differences in the component items; indeed, the majority of the items that appear on the OOC but not on the OCS occur on the postpartum subscale. The lack of similarity among the complication scales and the general lack of similarity between the complication and the optimality scales seem to be due to true differences in the specific items included on the scales.

The results of the analyses of the usefulness of these scales in predicting neonatal and infant outcome measures converge to indicate that in general, the complication scales are better predictors than the optimality scales. This holds true both for medical outcome measures that traditionally have been used to validate complication scales (e.g., gestational age, Apgar scores, neonatal status, and postnatal complications) and for measures with more behavioral relevance (e.g., scores on the Brazelton subscales and total scale, on the Carey Infant Temperament Questionnaire, and on the Bayley—Mental scale). The three complication scales (the UCNM, the HRPSS, and the RROS) predicted 29%, 29%, and 43% of the seven medical outcome measures and 27%, 7%, and 20% of the 15 behavioral outcome measures, respectively. The two optimality scales (the OOC and the OCS) predicted only 14% and 0% of the medical outcome measures and 13% and 7% of the behavioral outcome measures, respectively. Both the complication and the optimality scales were better predictors of medically relevant measures than of behaviorally relevant measures. This finding may reflect the medical science origins of the items included in the five scales.

It also appears that all five scales are better predictors of the neonatal outcome measures than of the infant outcome measures. These and other perinatal assessment scales have been found to be better predictors of neonatal outcomes than of infant outcomes in other studies as well (Bee *et al.,* 1982). Thus attempts to apply these scales to predicting behaviors in later infancy may be fruitless, since making such predictions seems to exceed the capabilities of these scales. To achieve accurate predictions of measures for later developmental periods, it may be necessary to reformulate the existing scales or to develop new ones.

Overall, the results suggest that complication scales may have a predictive advantage over optimality scales, because the three complication scales assessed in this study predicted a greater number and variety of outcome measures commonly used in predictive research with neonates and young infants. It is important to note that although the subjects in this study were generally healthy, all but three, nevertheless, had experienced multiple risk factors during the antepartum and/or intrapartum periods. It is likely that a study conducted on a less healthy sample would find that the subjects had experienced a greater number of different types of antepartum, intrapartum, and/or postpartum risk, and the results would be expected to differ from those obtained in this study.

Finally, the use of weighted scores as measures of perinatal risk, compared to the use of unweighted scores, produced some advantages in the correlations with the outcome measures. The differences in predictive validity between the complication scales and the optimality scales may be due to differences in the basis on which scores are assigned to risk conditions, with the differential weights assigned to risk conditions by the complications scales producing the stronger correlations with the outcome measures.

CHAPTER

5

Toward Developing a New Scale

In the previous two chapters, six perinatal risk scales were compared in order to answer questions regarding the similarity of the scores they generate. The abilities of the scales to predict a variety of maternal, neonatal, and infant outcome measures also were evaluated. Although some of the scales can predict many different types of outcome measures, none of the scales can predict all of the commonly used measures. In addition, the amount of variance accounted for by even the best scales is low, ranging from 5% to 14%. Clearly, these perinatal risk scales fall short, but it is unclear whether better scales can be created.

To explore the question of developing a better scale, I and my colleagues began a multistep research project in which we obtained data from three samples of women and their infants. In Step 1, analyses were run, item by item, on scores obtained from five of the six perinatal risk scales. The OOC (Prechtl) was not included because of the similarity of its items to those on the OCS (Littman & Parmelee), which was included. These analyses were used to identify the value of each item in predicting six different infant outcome measures. The six that were selected were chosen because they have often been used in medical and behavioral studies of predictive validity and in studies of infant and child development.

In Step 2, two types of scales were constructed, each of which was composed only of the items that were identified in Step 1 as predictive of one or more of the outcome measures. The predictive items were used to construct a general composite scale, composed of all predictive items, and six outcome-specific scales, each of which was composed only of items predictive of each single outcome measure.

In Step 3, data were obtained from a new sample of women and infants for use in comparison with data obtained earlier from a different sample of women and infants. The purpose of comparing the two subject samples was to determine if the predictive values obtained using the new composite scales would be reliable across samples and how the predictive validity of the new composite scales would compare to the predictive validity of the original scales.

STEP 1: IDENTIFYING THE PREDICTIVE ITEMS

The first step was to identify the specific items in the total pool of items from the five perinatal risk scales that would be included in the analyses. All of the items that were selected from the pool were those that were not redundant with other items in the pool. For example, if "toxemia in pregnancy" appeared on two scales but was weighted or defined differently on each, then two items were used. If, however, the weightings and the definitions were the same, only one "toxemia in pregnancy" item was used. A total of 268 nonredundant items were compiled from the pool of 303 items on the five perinatal risk scales. These 268 items were used, in subsequent item analyses, to identify the types of complications that could be used to predict specific outcomes.

The item analyses were designed to provide information on the interrelatedness of complications and outcomes. Some types of complications were known to be associated with specific types of outcomes. For example, teenaged mothers tend to have low birthweight and preterm infants; thus maternal age tends to cluster together with both birthweight and gestational age. The item analyses were to provide information to confirm what was known about the types of complications that cluster together with the outcome measures under study and to provide information on other complication–outcome clusters. These analyses, then, were used to identify items that might be reliably related to each outcome measure.

The item analyses were also designed to reveal which complications were not related to the outcome measures under study. The unrelated items could then be eliminated from further consideration, thus simplifying the scoring process. Since most of the items on the five perinatal risk scales had not previously been examined through such item analysis, it seemed likely that at least some of the items might not be predictive of the outcome measures. In addition, as Hobel (1980) has noted, because of changes in antepartum and intrapartum care and in the types of medical interventions that are possible, complications that once tended to result in specific types of perinatal risks might no longer be predictive of such risks. It also seemed possible that complication items might not be predictive of outcome measures for other reasons, such as the use of defining characteristics that were too narrow and that excluded most cases, the use of weighted scores that gave too little weight to one item relative to others, or a low incidence of a complication in the subject population under study, regardless of its defining characteristics and risk scores.

Discriminant function analyses were used for the item analyses because of our overall interest in determining whether the items would correctly classify the infants as having "normal" versus "abnormal" outcomes. In discriminant function analyses, the criterion measures (the dependent variables) are categorical (e.g., normal vs. abnormal), and subjects' scores on the individual items are used to determine the their classification on the outcome measures. For these analyses, data were obtained from the sample of 103 women and their infants described in Chapter 4. The women ranged in age from 15 to 38 years ($\bar{x}$ = 26.03 years). All delivered live infants, 25 by cesarean section (16 primary, 9 repeat). The infants' birthweights ranged from 2,353 to 5,215 grams ($\bar{x}$ = 3,472.4 grams), and their gestational ages, from 34 to 44 weeks ($\bar{x}$ = 39.7 weeks). The 1- and 5-minute Apgar scores ranged from 3 to 9 ($\bar{x}$ = 7.8) and from 7 to 10 ($\bar{x}$ = 8.9), respectively. Scores on the PNCS ranged from 0 to 4 points ($\bar{x}$ = 1.02). Neonatal status scores from the HRPSS ranged from 0 to 35 points ($\bar{x}$ = 2.62).

Data were obtained from medical records and demographic questionnaires and were used to score the 268 items. The data were also used to score the six outcome measures: birthweight, gestational age, 1- and 5-minute Apgar scores, scores on the PNCS, and neonatal status scores from the HRPSS. The scores on the outcome measures were used to categorize the subjects as normal or abnormal, using one of three different methods. The categorical system suggested by Apgar (1953) was used to classify scores on the Apgar scale: Scores greater than 7 at 1 minute and greater than 8 at 5 minutes were considered normal. For birthweight and gestational age, normal scores were those that fell within and around one standard deviation of the mean obtained with the study sample. For PNCS scores and HRPSS neonatal status scores, normal scores were those that were one standard deviation below the mean obtained with the sample. Scores considered abnormal for all measures were those that fell outside of the normal category. In analyses involving birthweight and gestational age, the abnormal category was further divided into "abnormal—high" and abnormal—low," since the end points of these measures were thought to represent different consequences for infant status.

For each outcome measure, individual antepartum and intrapartum items from the total pool of nonredundant items were entered into the discriminant function analysis in the order of their ability to discriminate between normal and abnormal outcome. Those items that resulted in the greatest increase in the overall multivariate *F* ratio for the test of differences between group centroids were entered first. Additional items were added by the analysis program until the *F* ratio reached nonsignificance or until all the items had been entered. A maximum of 50 steps was set for each discriminant analysis, which proved to be a sufficient number for completing the analysis. Items confounded with the outcome measures were deleted prior to analysis in order to avoid spuriously high correlations. For example, in analyses using birthweight as an outcome measure, items such as intrapartum estimates of fetal weight were deleted from the scale.

From these analyses, 108 items, or conditions, were identified as predictive of one or more outcome measures. These items and the outcome measures are shown in Table 5-1. The scale on which each item appears and the number of the item on the scale are shown in parentheses after each item name. Isolating these predictive items from the pool of 268 produced interesting results. Many of the items contained on the scales

TABLE 5-1. Conditions Identified as Predictive of Infant Outcome Measures

Condition	Apgar		Birthweight	Gestational age	PNCS	HRPSS neonatal status
	1-min	5-min				
Antepartum						
Abortions						
Habitual (B24)				×		
1, 2, 3+ (D05)	×			×	×	
Acute disorders/diseases						
Acute problems (C14)					×	
Hyperemesis (C20)		×			×	
Acute/chronic disorders (D11)	×	×		×		
Acute cystitis (B11)		×				
Viral disease (B38)		×		×		
Pulmonary disease (B45)			×	×		×
Flu (B46)						×
Age (in years)						
<16, <18 (E01)				×		×
<18, >30 (C04)			×			
<15, >35 (B37)			×			
<17 (A03)			×	×		
Anemia						
9–10.9 gm Hb (B48)		×			×	
<11 gm Hb (D20)	×	×				
<10 gm Hb (D32)		×		×		
Bleeding						
Spotting (B47)	×	×				
>20 wk (D35)						×

Blood pressure problems						
>140/90 (C18)		×	×			
Chronic disease/disorders						
Physical disorders (E06)	×					
Chronic disease (C16)			×		×	
Renal disease (B03)	×		×	×	×	×
Chronic hypertension (B02)						×
History of pyelitis (B06)			×			
Kidney disease (B09)		×				
Thyroid (B15)						×
Endocrine disorders (D17)	×					
Diabetes						
Family history of diabetes (B17)	×			×	×	×
Diabetes (D14)				×	×	×
Diabetes (B13)	×	×	×			
Drug abuse						
Chronic (C17)					×	
Excessive use of drugs (B42)			×			
Alcohol (B50)	×	×	×	×	×	×
Smoking < 1 pack/day (B49)						×
Drugs in pregnancy						
Chronic medication (E05)					×	×
In pregnancy (C15)				×		
Fertility						
Sterility (C08)	×	×		×		
Sterility (D19)				×		×
Gynecological problems						
Uterine malformation (B29)						×
Small pelvis (B33)					×	
Disproportion (C11)	×			×	×	

(continued)

Table 5-1. *(Continued)*

Condition	Apgar		Birthweight	Gestational age	PNCS	HRPSS neonatal status
	1-min	5-min				
Abnormal cervical cytology (B34)		×		×		×
Cervical problems (D25)	×	×				
Recurrent menstrual dysfunction (D18)	×	×	×			
Ovarian masses (D29)	×		×			
History of disease						
Cystitis (B10)	×					×
Toxemia (B12)						×
TB (B43)		×			×	
Eclampsia (B05)		×	×	×	×	
Parity						
Interval since last pregnancy (C09)		×	×	×		
Parity (C10)			×			
Parity (D04)					×	×
Prenatal care						
Categories of visits (A18)	×				×	
Prior premature infant						
Prior premature infant (C06, B21)			×			×
Prior low birthweight infant (A02)	×			×		
Rh problems						
Rh antagonism (C12)	×		×	×	×	
Rh sensitivity (B39)		×		×		
Rh problems (D21)		×				
Rh isoimmunization (A12)					×	×

Section (prior)						
Prior cesarean section (B23)					×	×
Prior cesarean section (D24)					×	
Socioeconomic factors						
Marital status (C03)		×	×			×
Marital status (D03)	×				×	
Race (D02)	×	×				
Stillbirth/neonatal death (prior)						
Stillbirth (C07)						×
Stillbirth (B19)			×			
Fetal death (D07)		×				
Neonatal death (D08)						×
Toxemia						
Mild (B08)			×			
Mild–severe (D30)			×			
Weight						
<100 or >200 lb (B44)		×				
Obese; adequate diet but malnourished (D22)		×				
Other pregnancy complications						
Surgery and accidents (A13)			×			
Amniocentesis (A16)				×	×	×
Intrapartum						
Abnormal presentation						
Not vertex (E10)						×
Breech (A08)					×	
Breech (B88)			×			
Prior malpresentations (D23)	×					
Amniotic fluid						
Turbid, bloody (E13)	×	×				

(continued)

TABLE 5-1. (*Continued*)

Condition	Apgar		Birthweight	Gestational age	PNCS	HRPSS neonatal status
	1-min	5-min				
Dark, meconium (B76)		×				
Meconium (D41)	×	×				
Cord problems						
Types (C33)			×			
Drugs in labor						
Analgesia (E16)				×		
Any drugs (C29)	×					
Medical induction (B65)					×	×
General anesthesia (B89)			×			
Fetal heart rate						
Low (E21)	×		×			
<100 or >160 beats/min (C32)						×
Bradycardia (B81)		×	×			
<115 or >165 beats/min (D42)	×					
Length of labor						
Long 1st or 2nd stage (E18)			×	×	×	
Short 1st or 2nd stage (E19)	×		×	×		
Duration, 1st stage (C26)	×		×	×		
Duration, 2nd stage (C27)			×	×		
Duration—short total (B66)					×	
Long 2nd stage (B63)					×	
Duration—long total (B62)	×	×				
Precipitous labor (B66)						×

Labor problems						
Labor complications (A09)						×
Delivery complications (A21)	×					
Dysfunction of labor (B58)		×				
Placenta problems						
Problems (E12)					×	
Infarction (C35)				×		
Premature rupture of membranes						
Premature rupture (E09)	×	×	×	×	×	×
>12 hr (B57)		×	×	×	×	
Premature rupture (A14)		×	×	×	×	
Section						
Planned/unplanned (E07)			×	×		×
Primary section (B67)	×					

Note. A = items from the UCNM; B = items from the HRPSS; C = items from the OCS; D = items from the MCHCI + LI; E = items from the RROS. From "Perinatal Risk Screening and Infant Outcome: Can Predictions Be Improved with Composite Scales" by V. Molfese, B. Thomson, B. Beadnell, M. Bricker, and L. Manion, 1987. *Journal of Reproductive Medicine, 32,* pp. 572–574. Copyright 1987 by the *Journal of Reproductive Medicine.* Reprinted by permission.

were not found to be predictive of any outcome measures. The number of nonpredictive items ranged from 24% to 67% of the total items on each scale. Given that the typical number of items on existing perinatal risk scales is 40, elimination of the nonpredictive items would reduce the number of items on the scales to between 13 and 30.

Of the 108 items that were identified as predictive, 75 pertained to antepartum complications and 33 to intrapartum complications. Interestingly, the proportion of antepartum items relative to intrapartum items was 69% to 31%. These percentages are similar to the 60%–40% and 70%–30% antepartum to intrapartum splits typically found on perinatal risk scales. It is also interesting to note from the presentation of items in Table 5-1 that there are 23 antepartum and 10 intrapartum categories. These numbers of categories are nearly identical to those constructed in Chapters 3 and 4 for items on the existing scales. That the predictive items distribute themselves broadly across a similar number of categories may support the validity of these categories in predicting outcome measures such as those used here.

Although the discriminant function analyses eliminated the nonpredictive items, some of the predictive items that remained appeared to be redundant. For example, duplicate items labeled "diabetes," "sterility," and "parity" are shown in Table 5-1. However, these apparently similar items differed from each other in the defining characteristics used to assess risk and in the weightings given to the items. In addition, different outcome measures were predicted by these seemingly redundant items. For example, diabetes (B13) predicted 1- and 5-minute Apgar scores and birthweight, whereas diabetes (D14) predicted gestational age, PNCS scores, and HRPSS neonatal status scores. Although these two items are similar, they differed in both definition and weighting.

Other examples of seemingly redundant items can also be found in the table. In each case, however, the items differed in weighting, in definition, or in both. In some cases, items had the same defining characteristics but were weighted differently; some of these items were also found to predict the same outcome measures. For example, both items labeled "prior

cesarean section" (B23 and D24) predicted PNCS scores. However, B23 had a weight of 5 points and D24 a weight of 30 points. In these cases, it appears that the items were so predictive that the specific weightings were unimportant above some minimum level.

Half of the individual predictive items were related to several different outcome measures. Of the predictive items, 51 (47%) predicted one outcome measure, 34 (31%) predicted two outcome measures, and 23 (21%) predicted three or more of the six outcome measures. Thus slightly more than 50% of the items predicted two or more outcome measures. The pattern of outcome measures predicted by specific items indicates that many items tend to be predictive of specific outcome measures rather than of outcome measures in general. For example, all the items pertaining to amniotic fluid problems were related to 1- and 5-minute Apgar scores, and all the maternal age items were related to birthweight, gestational age, and/or HRPSS neonatal status scores. None of the items on the table was predictive of all outcome measures.

STEP 2: CONSTRUCTING NEW COMPOSITE SCALES

The second step was to determine if the predictive items could be combined into scales that would yield scores with predictive values that were as good as, or better than, those obtained with existing scales.

The predictive items were used to construct two types of scales: a general composite scale and six outcome-specific composite scales. The general composite scale included all 108 predictive items identified by the item analyses in Step 1. It is similar to the perinatal risk scales from which it was derived in that it is designed to screen for a variety of outcome measures.

Each of the six outcome-specific scales was composed exclusively of items identified as predictive of one specific outcome measure. Thus the outcome-specific scale for birthweight contains only items predictive of birthweight, that for gestational age contains only items predictive of gestational age, and so forth. The numbers of items on the outcome-specific scales are remarkably similar: birthweight, 36 items; gestational age, 33 items; 1-minute Apgar, 32 items; 5-minute Apgar, 35 items; PNCS, 32 items; and HRPSS neonatal status subscale, 33 items.

STEP 3: ESTABLISHING RELIABILITY AND PREDICTIVE VALIDITY

The predictive values of the general composite scale and the outcome-specific composite scales were evaluated using data obtained from two samples of women and their infants. The purpose of the evaluation was to determine the accuracy of the scores generated by the composite scales in predicting each outcome measure. The first sample (Sample 1) consisted of 116 women and their infants who participated in a retrospective study in which data were obtained in the postpartum period. This sample of women and infants is described in Chapter 3.

The second sample (Sample 2) consisted of 96 women and their infants who were part of a prospective study of psychological traits and stress in pregnancy. The women were recruited during the 8th month of pregnancy, and perinatal risk data and outcome measures were obtained during the postpartum period. The women in this sample ranged in age from 17 to 40 years ($\bar{x}$ = 27.22 years). All delivered live infants, 17 by cesarean section (11 primary, 6 repeat). The infants' birthweights ranged from 2,466 to 4,706 grams ($\bar{x}$ = 3,484.3 grams), and their gestational ages ranged from 37 to 43 weeks ($\bar{x}$ = 39.8 weeks). The 1- and 5-minute Apgar scores ranged from 1 to 9 ($\bar{x}$ = 7.14) and from 6 to 10 ($\bar{x}$ = 8.65), respectively. Scores on the PNCS ranged from 0 to 4 points ($\bar{x}$ = .31). Neonatal status scores from the HRPSS ranged from 0 to 30 points ($\bar{x}$ = 4.75). Two of the infants were preterm and were placed in the special care nursery.

The predictive values of the general composite scale and the outcome-specific composite scales were tested using Pearson product–moment correlations and multiple regression analyses. The results of the correlational analyses are shown in Table 5-2. As can be seen, the Pearson correlations that

TABLE 5-2. Results of Correlational Analyses on Two Samples of Subjects

Sample	Birthweight	Gestational age	1-min Apgar	5-min Apgar	PNCS	HRPSS neonatal status subscale
General composite scale						
Sample 1	NS	– .23**	– .27**	– .21**	.23**	.38**
Sample 2	NS	NS	– .19*	– .18*	.17*	.42**
Outcome-specific composite scale						
Sample 1	– .22**	– .22**	– .20*	– .15*	.29**	.33**
Sample 2	NS	NS	– .18*	– .25**	.18*	.33**

Note. NS = not significant. For Sample 1, N = 116; for Sample 2, N = 96. From "Perinatal Risk Screening and Infant Outcome: Can Predictions Be Improved with Composite Scales" by V. Molfese, B. Thomson, B. Beadnell, M. Bricker, and L. Manion, 1987. *Journal of Reproductive Medicine, 32,* pp. 575. Copyright 1987 by the *Journal of Reproductive Medicine.* Reprinted by permission.

*p <.05.

**p < .01.

reached significance range from –.15 to .42. The strongest correlations for both subject samples were obtained for HRPSS neonatal status scores. The magnitudes of the correlations for the other outcome measures were, for both samples, quite similar.

The correlations obtained with the general composite scale and with the outcome-specific scales were compared with the correlations obtained in our previous studies with the five original perinatal risk scales. Table 5-3 shows Pearson product–moment correlations between scores on the original scales and the six outcome measures. The correlations that reached significance range from –.16 to .59. The correlations obtained with the composite scales, when compared with those obtained from the original scales, varied considerably across samples. For Sample 1, the correlations between the scores obtained on the original scales and the outcome measures were generally as large as, or larger than, the correlations obtained on the composite scales. For this sample, the original scales seem to have produced stronger correlations. However, for Sample 2, the correlations obtained using the composite scales were stronger and more often reached significance compared to the correlations produced using the original scales. The two samples apparently differed in terms of the risk conditions that were present in the subjects. These differences, together with differences between the items contained on the original scales and those on the composite scales, influenced the extent to which scale scores were systematically related to the outcome measures.

Shown in Table 5-4 are the results of the multiple regression analyses on the data obtained from both samples using scores from the general composite scale and the outcome-specific scales as predictors. In these analyses, the antepartum item scores were summed and entered in the equation first, followed by the intrapartum item scores.

Using the general composite scale scores, birthweight and 5-minute Apgar scores could not be predicted for Sample 1 or for Sample 2. Gestational age could be predicted for Sample 1 but not for Sample 2. One-minute Apgar scores, PNCS scores, and HRPSS neonatal status subscale scores could be predicted for both samples.

Table 5-3. Results of Correlations between Scores on the Original Scales and the Outcome Measures

Sample	Birthweight	Gestational age	1-min Apgar	5-min Apgar	PNCS	HRPSS neonatal status subscale
UCNM						
Sample 1	NS	− .21**	− .48**	− .45**	.53**	.59**
Sample 2	NS	NS	− .21*	.20*	.20*	.29**
OCS						
Sample 1	− .27**	− .33**	− .34**	− .24**	.57**	.52**
Sample 2	NS	.23**	NS	NS	NS	.19*
HRPSS						
Sample 1	NS	− .19*	− .30**	− .18*	.38**	.54**
Sample 2	NS	.27**	NS	NS	NS	.24**
MCHI + LI						
Sample 1	NS	− .17*	− .22**	− .20*	NS	.26**
Sample 2	NS	NS	NS	NS	.17*	.39**
RROS						
Sample 1	− .16*	− .25**	− .28**	− .18*	.57**	.53**
Sample 2	NS	.18*	− .24**	NS	NS	.20*

Note. NS = not significant. For Sample 1, $N = 116$, for Sample 2, $N = 96$.
*$p<.05$.
**$p<.01$.

TABLE 5-4. Results of Regression Analyses between Composite Scales and Outcome Measures

Sample	Birthweight	Gestational age	1-min Apgar	5-min Apgar	PNCS	HRPSS neonatal status subscale
			General composite scale			
Sample 1	NS	F = 3.10*	F = 3.10*	F = 2.98	F = 3.09*	F = 10.08**
		R = .22	R = .22	R = .20	R = .22	R = .42
Sample 2	NS	NS	F = 3.09*	F = 2.64	F = 6.56**	F = 11.09**
			R = .27	R = .23	R = .35	R = .44
			Outcome-specific composite scales			
Sample 1	F = 3.07*	F = 12.27**	F = 2.08	F = 7.29**	F = 5.39**	F = 7.94**
	R = .22	R = .42	R = .20	R = .35	R = .30	R = .36
Sample 2	NS	NS	F = 3.73*	F = 5.07**	F = 5.15**	F = 5.29**
			R = .27	R = .32	R = .23	R = .23

Note. NS = not significant. For Sample 1, N = 116; for Sample 2, N = 96. From "Perinatal Risk Screening and Infant Outcome: Can Predictions Be Improved with Composite Scales" by V. Molfese, B. Thomson, B. Beadnell, M. Bricker, and L. Manion, 1987. *Journal of Reproductive Medicine, 32,* p. 575. Copyright 1987 by the *Journal of Reproductive Medicine*. Reprinted by permission.

$^{*}p < .05$

$^{**}p < .01$.

Using the outcome-specific scale scores, birthweight and gestational age could be predicted only for Sample 1. One-minute Apgar scores could be predicted only for Sample 2. However, 5-minute Apgar scores, PNCS scores, and HRPSS neonatal status scores could be predicted for both samples.

Combining the predictive items into the two types of composite scales produced remarkably similar results. Within each sample, the outcome measures predicted by general composite scale scores were the same as those predicted by outcome-specific scale scores, with the exception of birthweight for Sample 1 and 5-minute Apgar scores for both samples, which would be predicted by the outcome-specific scale scores, and 1-minute Apgar scores for Sample 1, which could only be predicted by general composite scale scores. Additionally, for both types of composite scales, between 5% and 19% of the variance could be accounted for in the regression equations.

The performance of the composite scales in predicting the outcome measures can be compared to that of the original scales. Table 3-7 (see Chapter 3) shows the results of the multiple regression analyses that were run using scores from the original scales for the sample of 116 subjects (Sample 1). These results can be compared with those from the multiple regression analyses that were run using scores from the composite scales for the same subjects. Unfortunately, not all of the same outcome measures were included in the analyses, but both sets of analysis did use birthweight, gestational age, and 1- and 5-minute Apgar scores. Both the general composite scale and the outcome-specific scales predicted more of these outcome measures than were predicted by three of the five original scales. The two exceptions were the MCHCI + LI and the UCNM, both of which predicted scores on three of the four outcome measures and which were comparable with the results produced by the composite scales.

Of the four outcome measures used in both analyses of Sample 1, the MCHCI + LI (Table 3-7) did not predict gestational age, whereas the general composite scale (Table 5-4) did not predict birthweight. One outcome measure (5-minute Apgar scores) was not predicted by the general composite scale. Comparing the MCHCI + LI to the outcome-specific scales, the former did not predict gestational age, whereas the latter did not predict 1-minute Apgar scores. The UCNM predicted the same outcome measures as the general composite scale. The outcome-specific scales predicted one more outcome measure (birthweight) than the UCNM.

Since the overall amount of variance accounted for by the original scales and the composite scales is similar, and since both of the original scales are shorter, it might be argued that the original scales should be the scales of choice for use in predicting perinatal risk. Certainly, across a number of analyses (discussed in previous chapters), the performance of the MCHCI + LI was better than that of any of the other original scales, including the UCNM. However, 48% of the items on the MCHCI + LI and 60% of the items on the UCNM were not predictive of any of the six outcome measures used in our study. In contrast, all items on the general composite scale predicted at least one of the six outcome measures. Thus the general composite scale may provide an advantage over the original scales in the assessment of perinatal risk for obstetric populations that are similar to the one sampled in our study.

Although the composite scales were found to predict many of the six outcome measures, the amount of variance accounted for by the antepartum and intrapartum subscale scores was rarely higher than that produced by the original scales. Typically, the amount of variance was about the same for the composite and the original scales, though in some instances, less variance was accounted for by the new scales. We had hoped that the new scales would outperform the original scales. Clearly, additional refinement is needed before a distinct advantage may be demonstrated for the use of the composite scales.

The use of two subject samples permitted us to assess the composite scales both retrospectively and prospectively. The general scale and the outcome-specific scales consistently predicted one outcome measure more, and somewhat different outcome measures, for Sample 1 than for Sample 2. The cause of these differences is unclear. The two samples did differ in the manner in which subjects were selected: Those in Sample 1 were recruited during the postpartum period, and those in Sample 2, during pregnancy. Also, there were fewer subjects in

Sample 2 than in Sample 1. However, *post hoc t* tests for differences between the two samples were significant only for 1-minute Apgar scores ($t = 2.73$, $p < .01$) and neonatal status subscale scores ($t = 2.30$, $p < .05$). The composite scales did differ across samples in their ability to predict 1-minute Apgar scores, but there were no differences in their ability to predict neonatal status scores. There were no significant differences between samples for birthweight, gestational age, or 5-minute Apgar scores, but there were differences in the predictive values of these outcome measures between samples. The differences in results may be due to the inclusion, in the prospective sample, of subjects having subtle but important differences that might have been missed or not included in the retrospective sample, as has been traditionally argued.

SUMMARY

The combining of predictive items from the original perinatal risk scales into composite scales was found to result in the ability of the composite scales to predict a greater number of outcome measures than three of the five original scales. The new scales were similar in predictive ability to the MCHCI + LI and the UCNM. The total amount of variance accounted for by the composite scales was low (ranging from 5% to 18%) and still within the range of variance accounted for by the original scales. Further refinements in the weightings assigned to composite scale items may improve this measure.

CHAPTER
6

A Multivariate Model of Perinatal Risk

The preceding chapters have explored issues related to the effects of perinatal risk factors on measures of infant status at birth and of infant development during the first months of life. Although the origins of these risk factors have frequently been ascribed to physiological and medical conditions, other variables (e.g., psychological factors, stress, social processes) have also been identified as sources of perinatal risk. For example, anxiety, depression, and stressful life events in pregnancy are three phenomena that have received particularly intense scrutiny as sources of perinatal complications (Ascher, 1978; Ferreira, 1965; Grimm, 1967; McDonald, 1968). From the results of investigations of these variables, Chalmers (1982, 1984), Norbeck and Tilden (1983), Obayuwana, Carter, and Barnett (1984), and Warheit (1979) have proposed multivariate models that try to explain how several diverse variables interact with each other to produce perinatal complications, which, in turn, serve to influence maternal and infant perinatal outcomes. All of these models are based on the assumption that psychological and stress variables do not function independently to influence outcomes but rather work in synergy with physiological and medical variables. The purpose of these models has been to integrate the findings from past research and to provide a basis for new hypotheses concerning the influence on intrapartum events and infant outcome of psychological and stress variables that are present during the perinatal period.

In Chalmers's (1984) model, shown in Figure 6-1, pregnancy is seen as making a variety of demands on a woman. These demands give rise to the woman's perceptions of the stresses involved in being pregnant and of her emotional, cognitive, psychosocial, behavioral, and physiological abilities to cope with these stresses. Her efforts to cope with these stresses can result in a variety of responses, such as antepartum complications, social support seeking, the seeking of information on pregnancy and childbirth, and so forth. If the efforts in response to the stresses of pregnancy are perceived as being adequate, then the stresses are relieved. If, however, the responses are not perceived as adequate, various poor outcomes are hypothesized to result. In this model, poor perinatal outcomes are seen as arising from perceptions of past and present medical and obstetric characteristics. These perceptions give rise, in turn, to physiological responses to the present pregnancy and any antepartum complications.

A model similar to that of Chalmers and based on a stress model developed by Sarason (1979) was proposed by Norbeck and Tilden (1983). In this model, pregnancy produces a call to action that gives rise to variety of responses from the woman—for example, appraisals of social and personal resources available to deal with pregnancy, reactions to life events occurring before and during pregnancy, thoughts about herself and the tasks that are ahead. These responses are, in turn, appraised by the woman, and the appraisal leads to either a positive outcome of the pregnancy or a negative outcome, that is, a pregnancy with complications.

Warheit (1979) also proposed a stress model (Figure 6-2) in which life events are seen as making demands on the individual. The sources of the demands (i.e., the life events) are the individual's psychological and biological constitution, the culture, and the social environment. Various adaptive and nonadaptive screens develop from the individual's prior experience with these demands. Stress arises when the demands placed on the individual exceed his or her available coping resources. The outcomes of stress are symptoms, syndromes, and social dysfunctions.

Because these and other proposed multivariate models either have not been tested empirically or have been tested using only a subset of variables within the models, their validity is largely unknown. Recently, Molfese and colleagues (Molfese,

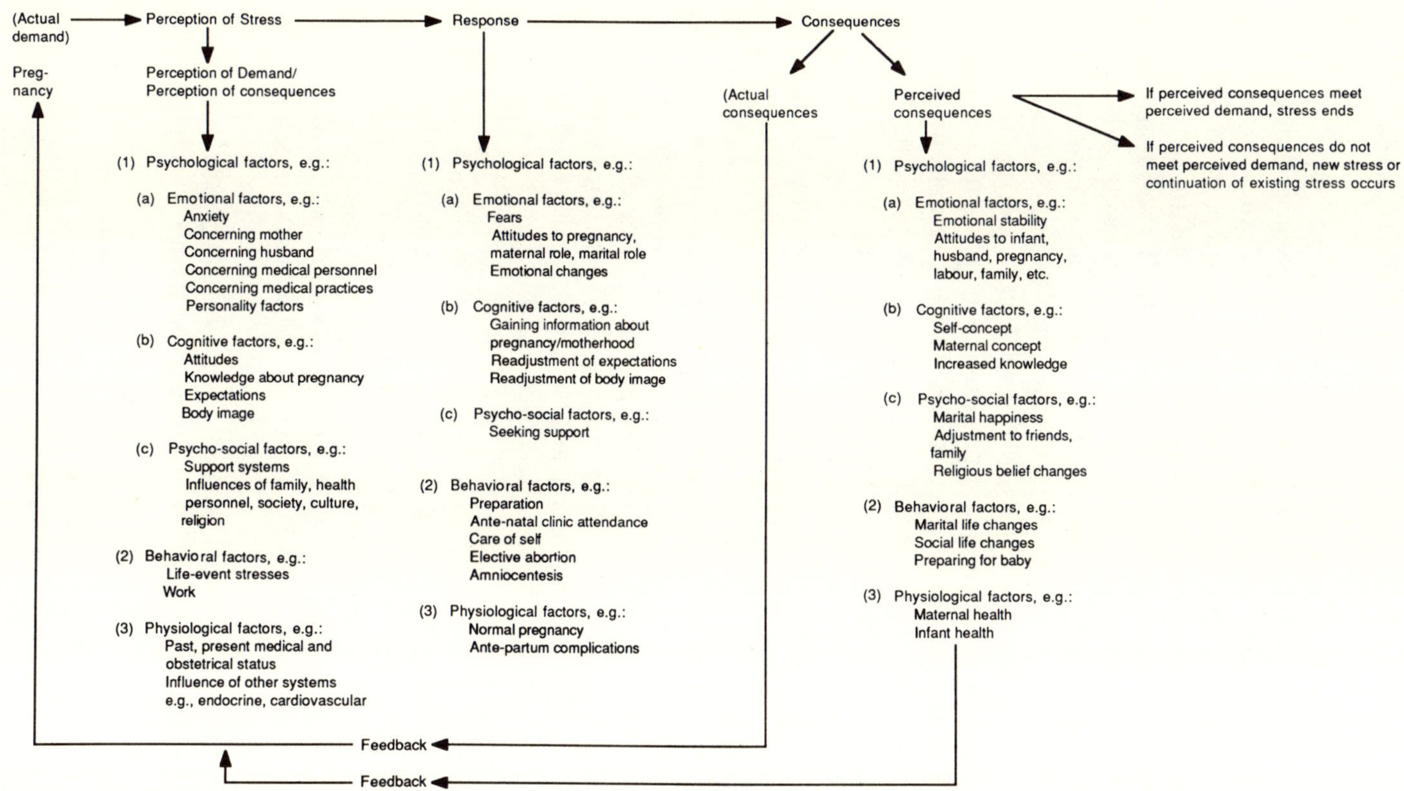

FIGURE 6-1. Chalmers's (1984) model of pregnancy. From "A Conceptualization of Psycho-social Obstetric Research" by B. Chalmers, 1984. *Journal of Psychosomatic Obstetrics and Gynecology, 3,* p. 19. Copyright 1984 by Elsevier Science Publishers B. V. Reprinted by permission.

Bricker, Manion, Beadnell, Yaple, & Moirs, 1987; Molfese, Bricker, Manion, Yaple, & Beadnell, 1987) proposed and empirically tested a multivariate model involving interactions among personality traits, stress during pregnancy, mediating variables, perinatal risks, and infant outcomes (see Figure 6-3). Two personality traits (anxiety and depression) and one measure of stress (life events stress) were used; the influence of these three variables on infant outcomes was seen as being moderated by attitudes toward pregnancy, internal versus external locus of control, and perception of available social supports. All of these variables have been identified in prior studies as influencing, to various degrees, infant outcomes. In addition, since various perinatal risks have been found to be associated with anxiety, depression, and stress in pregnancy, these

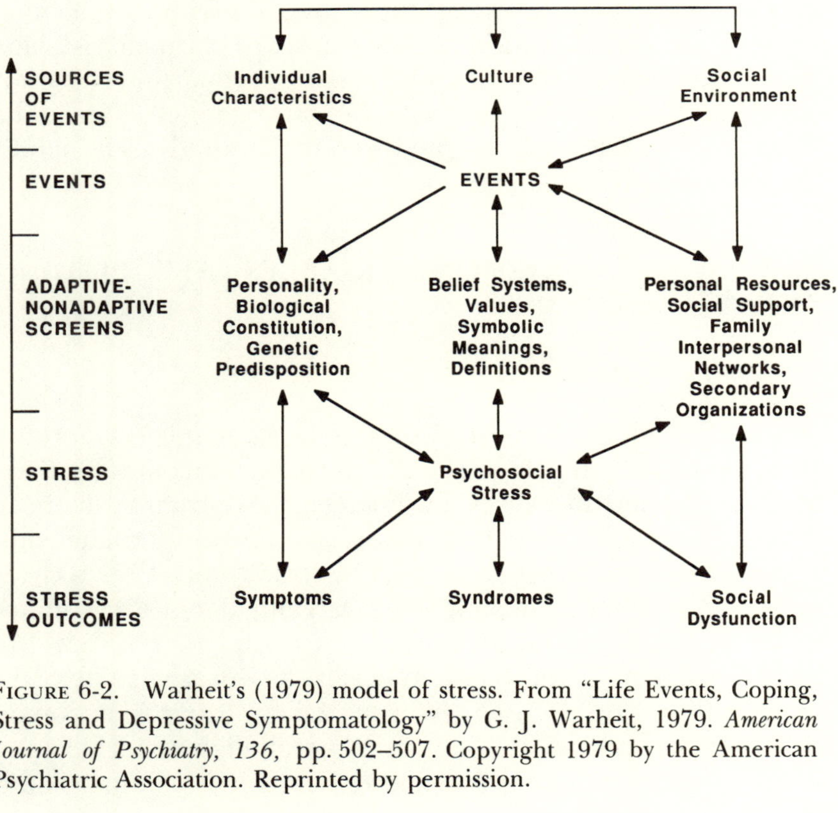

FIGURE 6-2. Warheit's (1979) model of stress. From "Life Events, Coping, Stress and Depressive Symptomatology" by G. J. Warheit, 1979. *American Journal of Psychiatry, 136,* pp. 502–507. Copyright 1979 by the American Psychiatric Association. Reprinted by permission.

Personality traits and stress	Mediating variables	Infant outcomes
Anxiety	Attitudes toward pregnancy	Apgar scores
Depression	Locus of control	HRPSS neonatal status scores
Life events stress	Perception of social supports	PNCS scores
	Perinatal risks	Birthweight
		Gestational age

FIGURE 6-3. A multivariate model of infant outcome.

risks are important variables to include in a model that seeks to account for the interrelationships of variables present during pregnancy that affect infant outcomes.

The next section reviews the literature on the variables of anxiety, depression, stress, attitudes toward pregnancy, locus of control, and social support as they pertain to perinatal risks and infant outcomes. Following this review is a report on the study conducted by Molfese, Bricker, Manion, Beadnell, Yaple, and Moirs (1987) that was designed to test the multivariate model shown in Figure 6-3.

REVIEW OF STUDIES ON VARIABLES AFFECTING INFANT OUTCOMES

ANXIETY

There is a long list of studies investigating the relationship between anxiety in pregnancy and perinatal outcomes. In these studies, higher measures of anxiety have commonly been found to be associated with a variety of poor perinatal outcomes (Burstein, Kinch, & Stern, 1974; Crandon, 1979; Davids & DeVault, 1962; Davids, DeVault, & Talmadge, 1961; Gunter, 1963; Klusman, 1975; McDonald & Christakos, 1963; McDonald & Parham, 1964; Shaw, Wheeler, & Morgan, 1970; Stanley, Soule, & Copans, 1979; Watson, Elliott, Rugg, & Borough, 1984; Zuckerman *et al.,* 1963). In general, high maternal anxiety in pregnancy has been found to be related to longer labor, greater use of analgesia and anesthesia in labor, premature birth, lower infant birthweight, and lower 5-minute Apgar scores. It has been somewhat difficult, however, to draw conclusions from these data, in part because of differences across studies in the type of anxiety measured and in the time during pregnancy when the measurement was obtained.

In working to refine the anxiety construct, Spielberger, Gorsuch, and Luschene (1970) described "anxiety" as involving a trait component and a state component. "Trait anxiety" is conceptualized as a relatively stable condition of anxiety proneness; it is an enduring personality characteristic that predisposes one to react in a specified manner and with predictable regularity. In contrast, "state anxiety" is a transitory condition of perceived tension arising in response to a specific situation; it refers to how a person feels at a given time.

Several researchers have used the state and trait constructs in their studies and have reported a link between level of state and/or trait anxiety and childbirth preparation, complications during pregnancy, labor and delivery events, neonatal status measures, and infant behavior (Beck *et al.,* 1980; Edwards & Jones, 1970; Gorsuch & Key, 1974; Lederman, Lederman, Work, & McCann, 1981; Lunenfeld, Rosenthal, Larholt, & Insler, 1984; Newton & Hunt, 1984; Norbeck & Tilden, 1983). The results across studies have generally shown that state anxiety varies considerably, depending on when measurement takes place. State anxiety is reported to reach a relatively moderate level during the last trimester of pregnancy, its highest level during labor, and its lowest level during the postpartum period (Astbury, 1980). Trait anxiety, on the other hand, has been found to be relatively constant across times of measurement. There have been reports that trait anxiety scores decline significantly during pregnancy compared to trait scores obtained during the postpartum period, but the changes in the trait anxiety scores have been smaller than the changes in scores reported for state anxiety (e.g., 4 points versus 11 points as reported by Lunenfeld *et al.,* 1984, and 3 points versus 8 points as reported by Astbury, 1980). Trait rather than state anxiety is presumed to be responsible for negative perinatal outcomes.

However, though high trait anxiety might be sufficient to produce perinatal complications, there is also evidence that state anxiety and anxiety related to life stress also contribute to perinatal complications (Gorsuch & Key, 1974; Carlson & LaBarba, 1979).

Depression

Unlike anxiety, depression has not been extensively investigated as a variable influencing perinatal outcome. Indeed, in Carlson and LaBarba's (1979) review of 57 studies of maternal emotionality in pregnancy and perinatal outcome, only one study is cited that included depression as a variable. Yet, depression was reported in *Lancet* as being "the most common neurotic disturbance in pregnancy" (Munro, 1984, p. 206). The literature reports prevalence rates for pregnant women ranging from 11% to 14%, depending on the criteria used to establish level of depression. Interestingly, depression has been associated, in the clinical literature, with persistent anxiety and/or stress, and a similar relationship has been reported in the obstetric literature as well. Norbeck and Tilden (1983) reported a high correlation (.73) between state anxiety and depression as measured by the Lubin Depression Adjective Checklist (Lubin, 1965). Tilden (1983) reported a correlation of .74 between depression and state anxiety and of .64 between depression and trait anxiety. Zajicek and Wolkind (1978) viewed depression and anxiety as representing a continuum of emotional reaction.

In addition to the preceding characteristics, depression has been reported to have several characteristics that are similar to those of anxiety. For example, some researchers have noted a trait aspect to depression, that is, that level of depression in pregnancy is predictive of level of depression during the postpartum period (Ballinger, 1982; Rees & Lutkins, 1971; Watson *et al.*, 1984; Warheit, 1979). Others, however, have questioned this notion by reporting evidence of antepartum depression or postpartum depression in various subjects but not both in the same subjects (Kumar & Robson, 1984; O'Hara, Neunaber, &

Zekoski, 1984). Depression has also been reported to influence perinatal outcomes in a manner similar to that shown by anxiety. High levels of depression are associated with more pregnancy complications, increased use of analgesia during labor, perinatal deaths, premature births, a higher incidence of neonatal resuscitations, and lower infant Apgar scores (Pilowsky & Sharp, 1971; Zax *et al.*, 1977; McDonald & Christakos, 1963; McDonald & Parham, 1964). Further, Zax *et al.* (1977) reported that it was the neurotic–depressed mothers who, when compared to schizophrenic or personality-disordered mothers, were found to have children with poor developmental scores during the first 3 years of life. Depression has also been found to be moderated by intervening variables, such as coping resources and social supports (Ballinger, 1982; Munro, 1984).

In sum, depression in pregnancy can be viewed as influencing perinatal outcomes in a manner similar to that shown by anxiety. The influence of depression seems to be moderated by the influences of intervening variables.

Stress

Stressful life events during or immediately prior to pregnancy have been characterized by some researchers as yet another form of anxiety (Chalmers, 1982). Several researchers have reported an association between anxiety and/or life stress and perinatal complications (Berkowitz & Kasl, 1983; Georgas, Giakoumaki, Georgoulias, Koumandakis, & Kaskarelis, 1984; Gorsuch & Key, 1974; Gunter, 1963; Jones, 1978; Newton & Hunt, 1984; Norbeck & Tilden, 1983; Rizzardo *et al.*, 1982). High stress as measured during pregnancy has been reported to be related to a variety of pregnancy complications (e.g., pre-eclampsia, hyperemesis, premature rupture of membranes, high blood pressure) and infant outcome measures (low birthweight, premature birth, low Apgar scores). Other researchers have reported associations between stressful life events and coping styles and/or social support systems (Chalmers, 1981; Nuckolls, Cassel, & Kaplan, 1972; Williams, Williams, Griswold, & Holmes, 1975; Norbeck & Tilden, 1983; Yamamoto & Kinney, 1976). Thus stressful life events seem to be influenced by anxiety and by the intervening variables that have been found to influence anxiety and depression.

Molfese, Bricker, Manion, Yaple, and Beadnell (1987) recently tested a multivariate model involving life events stress, intervening variables, and perinatal outcomes. In this prospective study, it was hypothesized that the influence of life events stress on intrapartum complications and infant outcomes would be moderated by adaptive factors such as attitudes toward pregnancy, locus of control, and perceived social support. The results of multiple regression analyses were interpreted as supporting the moderating role of the adaptive factors, since the ability of life events stress scores to predict the specific outcome measures was improved by the addition of mediating variables. Because many of the perinatal outcome measures could not be predicted from the life events stress measure alone, it was hypothesized that a more comprehensive model—one involving variables in addition to stress, such as anxiety and depression—might better illustrate the factors influencing perinatal complications.

Mediating Variables

Anxiety, depression, and stress, as single variables and in combination, have generally been found to be significant but weak correlates of perinatal outcomes. It appears that these variables interact with other, mediating variables that serve to modify the effects of the former, that is, to increase or decrease the influence of anxiety, depression, and stress on perinatal outcome. For example, depressed individuals with strong social support networks tend to have better perinatal outcomes than depressed individuals without such networks (Kumar & Robson, 1984). A wide variety of multidimensional intervening variables have been proposed by researchers. However, this review will focus only on the three variables that were incorporated in our multivariate model: attitudes toward pregnancy, locus of control, and perceived social support.

Attitudes toward Pregnancy

Although many different measures of attitudes toward pregnancy have been developed, the Maternal Attitude to Pregnancy Instrument (MAPI) (Blau, Welkowitz, & Cohen, 1964) is one of the few measures whose psychometric properties have been evaluated using factor analytic methods. The MAPI contains four subscales, which assess Acceptance of Pregnancy, Feelings of Well-Being, Active Participation in Pregnancy, and Special Fears. Women with complicated perinatal outcomes (e.g., prolonged labor and premature infants) have had MAPI scores indicating less positive attitudes toward pregnancy than those demonstrated by women without perinatal complications (Blau, Slaff, Easton, Welkowitz, & Cohen, 1963; Rosengren, 1961); in addition, highly anxious women tend to have less positive attitudes toward pregnancy (Zax, Sameroff, & Farnum, 1975). Interestingly, Zax *et al.* (1975) reported that there were no differences in MAPI scores among normal, schizophrenic, neurotic–depressed, and personality-disordered women. However, MAPI subscale scores, when combined with scores on life events stress, have been found to be predictive of scores on the intrapartum subscale of the High-Risk Pregnancy Screening System (HRPSS) and on induction-of-labor measures (Molfese, Bricker, Manion, Yaple, & Beadnell, 1987).

Locus of Control

Locus of control is a mediating variable that has not received much empirical study. It refers to measurements of a person's internal versus external orientation with regard to how reinforcement is controlled. People with an internal locus of control tend to feel more in control of their environments. In pregnancy, women with an internal locus of control might take more prenatal classes, attempt to provide better prenatal environments for their infants, and be more aware of changes that occur during their pregnancies. People with an external locus of control feel more at the mercy of their environments. Pregnant women with an external locus of control might be less involved in, and less prepared for, pregnancy. An interaction between locus-of-control measures and perinatal outcome measures has been discussed by several researchers (Grimm, 1967; O'Connell, 1983; Chalmers, 1983), but actual results from these studies have not been reported. Molfese, Bricker, Manion, Yaple, and Beadnell (1987) have reported that locus of control, when combined with scores on life events stress, MAPI subscale scores, and/or perceived social support scores, was found to be predictive of intrapartum scores on the Maternal–Child Health Care Index (MCHCI) and the Labor Index (LI), use of analgesia in labor, presence of meconium, and 1- and 5-minute Apgar scores.

Social Support

Social support has been identified by several researchers as a mediating variable that moderates the effects of stress on perinatal outcome (Nuckolls *et al.,* 1972; Norbeck & Tilden, 1983; Tilden, 1983; Barrera & Balls, 1983). Norbeck and Tilden (1983) reported that social support interacted with life stress to influence measures of emotional disequilibrium in pregnancy. Others (Nuckolls *et al.,* 1972; Barrera & Balls, 1983) have reported that life stress in the presence of strong social supports was related to positive pregnancy outcomes.

Recently, Smilkste (1984) proposed a biopsychosocial model of pregnancy complications. The biomedical risks (e.g., perinatal risks) and the psychosocial risks (e.g., measures of social support) were found to be negatively related to each other. Women with high biomedical risks were dissatisfied with their available social supports. Further, whereas biomedical risks were found to be unrelated to intrapartum or postpartum complications, psychosocial risks were found to be related to both types of complications. The lack of a relationship between the biomedical risks and the intrapartum and postpartum complications may have been due to the use by the study of a basically normal population.

In considering measures of social support, Kumar and Robson (1984) noted that the *perception* of social support, rather than the presence of such support, was the variable of importance. Social support may be present, but it if is not seen as being supportive, it will not play an important role. Molfese, Bricker, Manion, Yaple, and Beadnell (1987) found that perception of social support was a stronger predictor of the use of analgesia in labor and of infant birthweight than life events stress in regression equations combining the two variables.

Perinatal Complications

The role of perinatal complications in influencing perinatal outcomes has not been extensively examined in the published studies on personality and stress. Indeed, the primary focus of these studies has been on personality, stress, and intervening variables, with little attention having been paid to the perinatal complications that arise in response to, or along with, the variables under study. Most of these studies have tended to use standardized or well-known measures of personality, stress, and intervening variables, but instead of established measures of perinatal complications, they have often used a collection of study-specific complications. In some studies, the perinatal complications used were obtained from obstetric textbooks (e.g., Georgas *et al.,* 1984), and in other studies, they were simply those that were found to be present in the study sample (e.g., Gorsuch & Key, 1974). In studies where the subjects were categorized as "normal" or "abnormal," the assignment was based on the presence of any complication, regardless of severity (e.g., Nuckolls *et al.,* 1972; Rizzardo *et al.,* 1982), or on the judgment of a physician (Burstein *et al.,* 1974; Georgas *et al.,* 1984). Because of the differences across studies in how perinatal complications have been measured, it is difficult to compare the reported results.

Despite the differences across studies in the measures of perinatal complications, anxiety, depression, and stress have generally been found to be related to a variety of these complications. These findings, together with previous findings that perinatal complications influence maternal and infant outcomes, can be used as the basis for formulating a model in which a chain of events occurs. Within this chain, personality, stress, and intervening variables interact with perinatal complications to influence maternal and infant outcomes. It is important to determine whether the use of more standardized measures of perinatal complications would provide a fuller picture than has been provided by past research of the role of each variable in influencing maternal and infant outcomes.

In the study described in the next section, the outcome-specific perinatal risk scales described in Chapter 5 were used to quantify antepartum and intrapartum risk for infants. Since outcome-specific scales for predicting maternal outcomes have not yet been developed, the MCHCI (Nesbitt & Aubry, 1969) and the LI (Aubry & Pennington, 1973) were used to quantify antepartum and intrapartum risk for mothers. These indexes have been found to be useful in predicting a variey of outcome measures within the type of obstetric population from which the subject sample for this study was drawn (Molfese *et al.*, 1985; Molfese, Bricker, Manion, Yaple, & Beadnell 1987).

Although measures of perinatal complications have, in previous studies, frequently been treated as independent variables, they tend to be interrelated. That is, the presence of one perinatal complication tends to be associated with the presence of a variety of other complications (Parmelee *et al.*, 1976; Littman & Parmelee, 1978). Thus, in our study, scales containing a diversity of risk conditions, rather than a measure of a single risk condition, were used as measures. Each of the outcome scales is composed of a variety of specific complications and can be used for obtaining summary scores on perinatal risk. For purposes of comparison, eight individual measures of complications were also used, to determine what specific intrapartum and infant measures were related to the predictor variables.

STUDY OF THE MULTIVARIATE MODEL

The study described here was conducted by Molfese, Bricker, Manion, Beadnell, Yaple, and Moirs (1987). In this study, an attempt was made to test the multivariate model using personality traits, life events stress, mediating variables, perinatal complications, and perinatal outcomes. The test of the model involved several different steps, which are discussed under the Results section.

Characteristics of the Sample

The sample was drawn from groups of women who were contacted in their eighth month of pregnancy through obstetricians or prenatal classes. Those who volunteered to participate and who completed a series of questionnaires were included as subjects.

Data were obtained from 133 women and their infants. The women ranged in age from 16 to 40 years ($\bar{x}$ = 27.3 years). All delivered live infants, 28 by cesarean section (20 primary, 8 repeat). The infants' birthweights ranged from 2,466 to 4,833 grams ($\bar{x}$ = 3,518.39 grams). Gestational ages of the infants ranged from 37 to 43 weeks ($\bar{x}$ = 39.88 weeks). Their 1- and 5-minute Apgar scores ranged from 1 to 9 points ($\bar{x}$ = 7.24) and from 6 to 10 points ($\bar{x}$ = 8.71), respectively. Other characteristics of the women and their infants that were used as variables in the analyses are shown in Tables 6-1 and 6-2, respectively.

Measures

In their eighth month of pregnancy, the women completed a series of questionnaires: the Beck Depression Inventory (Beck, Ward, Mendelson, Mock, & Erbaugh, 1961); the state and trait portions of the State–Trait Anxiety Inventory (STAI) (Spielberger *et al.*, 1970), the PERI Life Events Scale (Dohrenwend, Krasnoff, Askenasv, & Dohrenwend, 1978), the Rotter Internal–External Locus of Control (I–E) Scale (Rotter, Chance, & Phares, 1972), the MAPI (Blau *et al.*, 1964), and the Perceived Social Support Inventory (Vaux, 1982). The means, standard deviations, and ranges for these measures are shown in Table 6-3.

The medical records of subjects were used to obtain data

TABLE 6-1. Descriptive Statistics on Maternal Characteristics and Outcome Measures

Characteristic	Outcome measure
Parity	HRPSS intrapartum risk
Nulliparas ($N = 62$)	Mean = 8.29 points
Primiparas ($N = 71$)	SD = 9.29 points
Employment	Range = 1–60 points
Employed ($N = 92$)	Length of 1st-stage labor
Unemployed ($N = 41$)	Mean = 524.79 min
Marital status	SD = 327.97 min
Single ($N = 5$)	Range = 45–1,650 min
Married ($N = 128$)	Length of 2nd-stage labor
Education	Mean = 56.28 min
Less than high school graduate ($N = 5$)	SD = 58.57 min
High school graduate ($N = 26$)	Range = 5–315 min
Some college ($N = 28$)	Anesthesia
College graduate ($N = 53$)	None ($N = 96$)
Postgraduate ($N = 21$)	Less than general ($N = 19$
Race	More than general ($N = 18$)
White ($N = 129$)	Analgesia
Nonwhite ($N = 4$)	None ($N = 91$)
Income	Less than 50 mg ($N = 15$)
Under $5,000 ($N = 3$)	More than 50 mg ($N = 27$)
$5,000–10,000 ($N = 12$)	
$10,000–15,000 ($N = 14$)	
$15,000–20,000 ($N = 21$)	
$20,000–25,000 ($N = 15$)	
$25,000–30,000 ($N = 17$)	
$30,000–35,000 ($N = 9$)	
Over $35,000 ($N = 39$)	
No information ($N = 3$)	

on events during pregnancy, labor, and delivery and on the postnatal status of the infants. The use of standardized antepartum, intrapartum, and postpartum medical record forms that were utilized at the hospital where all the subjects delivered their infants reduced the possibility of missing or incomplete medical information. Medical records data were used to score the following six outcome-specific scales (described in Chapter 5): birthweight, gestational age, 1- and 5-minute Apgar scores, scores on the Postnatal Complications Scale (PNCS), and neonatal status scores from the HRPSS. The items on each outcome-specific scale were grouped into antepartum and intrapartum subscales. The medical records data were also used

TABLE 6-2. Descriptive Statistics on Infant Outcome Measures

Outcome measure	Mean	*SD*	Range
Birthweight	3,518.39 gm	437.14 gm	2,466–4,833 gm
Gestational age	39.88 wk	1.34 wk	0–20 wk
1-minute Apgar	7.24	1.66	1–9
5-minute Apgar	8.71	0.62	6–10
PNCS	2.53 points	4.99 points	0–20 points
HRPSS neonatal status	2.53 points	4.99 points	0–20 points

to score the MCHCI and the LI. The means, standard deviations, and ranges for these measures are shown in Table 6-3.

The individual outcome measures that were used to evaluate the multivariate model were measures of labor events and infant status that are frequently used in studies of perinatal complications. The labor event measures were length of first-stage labor, length of second-stage labor, amount of analgesia, amount of anesthesia, and a summary score on intrapartum risk that was derived from scores on the intrapartum items of the HRPSS. The infant outcome measures were birthweight; gestational age; 1- and 5-minute Apgar scores; and summary scores on infant status obtained from PNCS scores and from scores on the neonatal status subscale, a group of 13 postnatal status items (prematurity, resuscitation at birth, fetal anomalies, feeding problems, respiratory distress syndrome, meconium aspiration syndrome, congenital pneumonia, anomalies of the respiratory system, apnea, transient tachypnea, hypoglycemia, jitteriness or hyperactivity with specific causes, and hyperbilirubinemia) taken from the HRPSS that characterize common neonatal complications. Descriptive statistics for these outcome measures are shown in Tables 6-1 and 6-2.

RESULTS

The usefulness of the multivariate model in predicting measures of maternal and infant outcomes was evaluated in several different steps. In an effort to reduce the total number of predictor variables, anxiety, depression, stress, and the mediating variables were analyzed using principal components factor

TABLE 6-3. Descriptive Statistics on Personality, Stress, and Mediating Variables

Measure	Mean	*SD*	Range
Personality–stress measures			
Beck Depression Inventory	8.5	4.48	1–23
STAI—State portion	33.21	9.00	20–69
STAI—Trait portion	36.45	8.90	19–64
PERI LIfe Events Scale	1,054.62	869.80	182–4,471
Measures of mediating variables			
Rotter I–E Scale	10.02	3.59	2–21
MAPI			
Acceptance of Pregnancy	49.92	9.64	2–70
Feelings of Well-Being	22.48	3.97	3–32
Active Participation in Pregnancy	9.76	2.08	5–15
Special Fears	25.39	4.07	15–37
Total score on Perceived Social Support Inventory	44.73	8.79	24–77
MCHCI antepartum risk	29.21	28.44	0–245
LI intrapartum risk	12.63	17.92	0–60
Outcome-specific antepartum risk			
Gestational age	18.45	17.27	0–104
1-minute Apgar	12.40	11.42	0–53
5-minute Apgar	16.93	18.02	0–73
PNCS	23.71	18.40	0–100
HRPSS neonatal status	18.99	17.07	0–107
Outcome-specific intrapartum risk			
Gestational age	9.89	13.55	0–54
1-minute Apgar	17.46	21.65	0–103
5-minute Apgar	13.59	18.62	0–96
PNCS	16.50	20.28	0–93
HRPSS neonatal status	13.68	17.10	0–66

analyses. The first analysis focused on the measures of anxiety, depression, and stress. One factor, Personality, had an eigenvalue of 2.35 that accounted for 58.8% of the variance. The variables of state anxiety, trait anxiety, and depression all loaded on the Personality factor, and the variables had similar factor loadings (.85, .89, and .82, respectively). Life events stress also loaded on the Personality factor but with a lower factor loading (.42).

The mediating variables were analyzed in a separate factor analysis. Three factors with eigenvalues of 1.65, 1.33, and 1.06, respectively, were produced: the first factor, Pregnancy Feelings, accounted for 27.4% of the variance, with loadings from the variables Special Fears (.85) and Feelings of Well-Being (.84) from the MAPI; the second factor, Pregnancy Acceptance, accounted for 22.2% of the variance, with loadings from the variables Acceptance of Pregnancy (.84) and Active Participation in Pregnancy (–.67) from the MAPI; the third factor, Locus of Control/Support, accounted for 18% of the variance, with loadings from the variables locus of control (.87) and the total score from the Perceived Social Support Inventory (.60).

Subsequent analyses were computed using scores on the four factors identified through the factor analyses. These scores, plus scores on the perinatal risk scales, were used in Pearson product–moment correlations. The correlations were computed in order to determine the relationship between the personality, stress, and mediating variables and the outcome measures. The correlations are shown in Table 6-4. The significant *r*'s, ranging from .15 to .59, are generally low. These low correlations are similar to those reported by other researchers and support the belief that the personality and stress variables do not directly influence perinatal outcomes.

The usefulness of the predictor variables in predicting scores on the specific outcome measures was examined using multiple regression and discriminant function analyses. The multiple regression analyses were used to predict three intrapartum outcome variables—HRPSS intrapartum risk scores, length of first-stage labor, and length of second-stage labor—and six infant outcome variables—birthweight, gestational age, 1-minute Apgar scores, 5-minute Apgar scores, PNCS scores, and HRPSS neonatal status scores. Because the intrapartum outcome measures of anesthesia and analgesia involved categorical data, discriminant function analyses were used to test predictions with those measures. The categories used in these analyses are shown in Table 6-1. Because of the large number of variables involved in the overall model, the number of regression and discriminant function models that could be tested was large. Thus, for each outcome measure, we analyzed (1) the full model, containing all the predictor variables (Per-

TABLE 6-4. Correlation of Anxiety, Depression, Stress, Mediating Variables, Pregnancy Complications, and Outcome Measures

	Infant outcome measures					Maternal outcome measures				
	Gestational age	1-min Apgar	5- min Apgar	PNCS	HRPSS neonatal status	Anesthesia	Analgesia	Stage-1 labor	Stage-2 labor	Intrapartum risk
Personality	.16	.03	−.04	−.08	−.18	.08	.19	.05	−.19	.03
State anxiety	.08	.04	−.03	−.06	−.05	.04	.12	.10	−.20	.01
Trait anxiety	−.05	−.02	.04	−.07	−.08	.01	.13	.09	−.18	−.03
Depression	.18	.14	.04	−.08	−.01	.10	.09	.01	−.13	.07
Life events stress	.08	−.01	−.01	.01	.14	.08	.19	.11	−.16	−.05
Pregnancy Feelings	.14	−.10	−.15	−.03	.01	−.03	−.01	−.15	.10	.01
Special Fears	.01	−.10	−.08	−.04	.03	−.08	−.04	−.06	.06	−.11
Feelings of Well-Being	.11	.04	.01	−.01	.06	−.07	−.10	−.15	.08	−.03
Pregnancy Acceptance	−.06	.04	−.01	−.17	−.16	−.12	.01	−.01	−.09	−.06
Acceptance of Pregnancy	−.08	.03	.07	−.09	−.05	−.04	−.04	−.05	−.03	−.05
Active Participation	.03	−.03	.06	.09	−.02	.20	−.03	.07	.08	.07
Locus of Control/Support	−.03	−.21	−.27	.04	.10	−.18	.07	−.09	.01	−.08
Locus of control	.01	−.25	−.28	.09	.12	−.02	.09	−.15	.04	.04
Perceived social support	−.02	.04	−.04	−.11	.10	.01	.02	.09	−.12	.13
Perinatal risk scales										
MCHCI—antepartum	.01	.01	−.01	.12		.23	.23	.31	.12	.29
LI—intrapartum	.14	−.22	−.22	.12		.23	.25	.18	.29	.59

Outcome-specific risk scales					
Gestational age—antepartum	.13				
Gestational age—intrapartum	.35				
1-min Apgar—antepartum		.12			
1-min Apgar—intrapartum		−.27			
5-min Apgar—antepartum			−.13		
5-min Apgar—intrapartum			−.34		
PNCS—antepartum				.19	
PNCS—intrapartum				.03	
HRPSS neonatal status—antepartum					.16
HRPSS neonatal status—intrapartum					.18

Note. All correlations > .15 are significant ($p < .05$).

sonality, Pregnancy Feelings, Pregnancy Acceptance, Locus of Control/Support, and pregnancy complications), and (2) models composed only of subsets of the variables.

Table 6-5 presents the results of the multiple regression analyses. Although a number of equations were found to be significant, only the equations that best predicted each outcome measure are shown in the table. As can be seen, combinations of the Personality and/or mediating factors with specific perinatal risk scale scores produced significant equations for eight of the nine outcome measures analyzed. (Birthweight could not be predicted by the predictor variables and thus was not included in the table.) The multiple R values produced by the equations exceeded the simple r for all outcome measures.

In the discriminant function analyses for analgesia, there were three groups (no analgesia, less than 50 milligrams, and more than 50 milligrams) to be discriminated. Personality (r = .74), MCHCI (r = .54), and LI (r = .80) were used to discriminate among the groups. The level of chance classification was 33.33%, and the classification accuracy 53.19% (z = 4.21, $p < .001$). For anesthesia, there were three groups (no anesthesia, less than general, more than general) to be discriminated. Locus of Control/Support (r = .90), MCHCI (r =

TABLE 6-5. Results of Regression Analyses on Maternal and Infant Outcome Measures

Measures and variables	Beta	F	R	R^2
	Maternal outcome measures			
Length of 1st-stage labor		5.85**	.33	.11
Pregnancy Feelings	−.16			
MCHCI—antepartum	.03			
LI—intrapartum	.22			
Length of 2nd-stage labor		3.33**	.29	.08
Personality	−.24			
LI—intrapartum	.22			
HRPSS intrapartum risk		11.32**	.67	.46
Personality	.12			
Pregnancy Feelings	.03			
Pregnancy Acceptance	−.04			
Locus of Control/Support	−.02			
MCHCI—antepartum	.32			
LI—intrapartum	.54			

(*continued*)

TABLE 6-5. (*Continued*)

Measures and variables	Beta	*F*	*R*	R^2
Infant outcome measures				
Gestational age		8.93**	.50	.25
Personality	.06			
Pregnancy Feelings	.24			
Gestational age—intrapartum	.43			
1-minute Apgar		7.38**	.34	.12
Locus of Control/Support	−.24			
1-minute Apgar—intrapartum	−.27			
5-minute Apgar		8.19**	.43	.18
Pregnancy Feelings	−.10			
Locus of Control/Support	−.27			
5-minute Apgar—intrapartum	−.31			
PNCS		4.62**	.28	.08
Pregnancy Acceptance	−.14			
PNCS—antepartum	.23			
HRPSS neonatal status		2.86**	.34	.12
Personality	−.13			
Pregnancy Acceptance	−.16			
HRPSS neonatal status—antepartum	−.20			
HRPSS neonatal status—intrapartum	.10			

*$p < .05$.
**$p < .01$.

.70), and LI ($r = .58$) were used to discriminate among the groups. The level of chance classification was 33.33%, and classification accuracy 63.03% ($z = 6.81$, $p < .001$).

CONCLUSIONS

The results of this study can be used to discuss several key issues pertaining to the effects on perinatal outcome of anxiety, depression, and stress in pregnancy; of the mediating variables of pregnancy attitudes, locus of control, and perception of social supports; and of pregnancy complications. The interrelationships of these variables indicated that anxiety, depression, and stress in pregnancy, though weakly related to the outcome measures, did predict, in combination with the mediating variables, some of the outcome measures. Length of second-stage labor, HRPSS intrapartum risk scores, infant gestational age, and HRPSS neonatal status scores were predicted from combinations of the Personality factor scores with scores on one or more of the mediating factors. For the other outcome measures, combinations of the mediating factor scores and perinatal complications scores produced the best predictions; the Personality factor scores were not significant correlates, or predictors, of these other measures. It appears that while portions of the multivariate model are useful for characterizing the relationships between the predictor variables and some of the outcome measures, the full model is not useful in predicting *all* measures.

The relationships between anxiety, depression, stress, and the mediating variables on the one hand and the outcome measures on the other were generally weaker than the relationships between the measures of perinatal complications and the outcome measures. This was true both in the correlational analyses, when individual measures of these variables were used, and in the regression and discriminant function analyses, when these measures were combined into factors (Personality, Pregnancy Feelings, Pregnancy Acceptance, and Locus of Control/Support). Perinatal complication scores had stronger simple correlations for seven of the ten outcome measures and heavier beta weights for all eight outcome measures for which significant regression equations were obtained. Perinatal complication scores also had stronger canonical correlations in one of the two discriminant function analyses.

These findings are important, because although many studies have examined the influence of anxiety, depression, stress, and the mediating variables on perinatal outcome, few have reported the specific contributions of these variables to the prediction of perinatal outcome measures. Interestingly, Chalmers (1984), Warheit (1979), and Obayuwana *et al.* (1984) all include pregnancy or physiological complications during pregnancy as a variable in their models of obstetric complications, but no studies have tested these complete models. Considering these models, it makes sense that perinatal complications would be more predictive of perinatal outcome than would the other variables, because perinatal complications are viewed as physiological responses to anxiety, depression, and stress and, as such, are mediators of perinatal outcome. Thus anxiety, depression, and stress are not thought to directly effect perinatal outcome. Other variables also serve mediating roles, but based on the results of our study, they are not as important as perinatal complications in determining outcome.

The low correlations between the anxiety, depression, stress, and mediating variables and the outcome measures may be due to the ranges of scores on these measures that were obtained from this particular sample of subjects. The subjects in our study were not selected for specific traits or characteristics, unlike subjects in many of the previously published studies. Although the scores that were obtained from our subjects did show a considerable range and did contribute toward the prediction of the outcome measures, there may have been fewer subjects with scores at the extreme ends of the range than might have been the case if subjects with characteristics outside of the norm had been sampled. If anxiety, depression, stress, and mediating variables influence outcome, then data obtained from subjects with extreme scores would be expected to exhibit more of the anticipated consequences than data obtained from subjects with normal scores. The lack of consistency in the literature concerning the effects on perinatal outcome of anxiety, depression, stress, and various mediating variables might reflect the degree to which the subjects sampled had those characteristics.

The results using the different measures of perinatal complications were interesting. In analyses designed to predict the infant outcome measures, the inclusion of outcome-specific scales or composite scales produced stronger equations than did the inclusion of the MCHCI or the LI. The different results might be due to differences in the specific items and in the item weightings on the outcome-specific and composite scales. Interestingly, only individual subscales from the outcome-specific scales were included in the strongest equations in predicting gestational age, 1- and 5-minute Apgar scores, and PNCS scores. However, for the HRPSS neonatal status scores, only the antepartum and intrapartum composite scales were strong predictors. It is not clear why these differences were found, but they could indicate that it might be necessary to further refine the outcome-specific scale for the HRPSS neonatal status scores.

In summary, the results of this study generally support our proposed multivariate model. With the exception of birthweight, which could not be predicted from combinations of the predictor variables, all of the outcome measures could be predicted from combinations of anxiety, depression, stress, or mediating variables and pregnancy complication scores. The results support the notion that these variables do not function independently in influencing outcome but work in synergy, since the multivariate analyses produced stronger predictive results than did simple correlations.

CHAPTER

7

A Reconsideration of Risk and Risk Assessment

Perinatal risk assessment has been presented in the preceding chapters in terms of the current state of the art. By far, the majority of current approaches are based on the traditional view that complications that increase the risks for poor perinatal outcomes can be identified and that the risks can then be minimized through therapeutic interventions, thus maximizing the perinatal outcomes. A number of perinatal risk scales have been developed on the basis of this traditional view. Each of these scales contains a variety of antepartum, intrapartum, and postpartum complications that are known or thought to negatively influence perinatal outcomes. A score, often arbitrarily weighted, is assigned to each complication as a means of quantifying the risk associated with it.

Although the scales have all been shown to be effective in identifying high-risk pregnancies, none has achieved the goal of being simple, reliable, and cost efficient (i.e., having low specificity and high sensitivity). High expectations remain concerning improvements that could be made in these scales. There is hope (1) that the scales can be improved on the basis of new findings in gynecology, obstetrics, and the behavioral sciences as they become available; (2) that the scales can be more closely tailored to fit the complications found in the specific obstetric populations to which the scales will be applied; and (3) that the scales scores will have predictive value not only for the perinatal period but for later developmental periods as well.

In an effort to expand the concept of risk assessment as it is applied to perinatal risk scales, this chapter explores several issues that are basic to the overall notion of "risk assessment."

Risk assessments are important components in a variety of decision-making tasks that involve issues as diverse as environmental safety, career development, and drug therapy. The perception of risk and the approaches taken to risk assessment in fields outside of obstetrics differ considerably. A consideration of these differences in perception and approach might provide new insights that would be useful in a reconsideration of perinatal risk. Wilson and Crouch (1987) have presented an introduction to risk assessment that includes issues pertaining to risk and uncertainty, risk estimation based on historical data, risk value versus certainty of information, and expression of risks. Each of these issues will be discussed here and will be related to perinatal risk.

According to Wilson and Crouch, the function of risk assessment is not to make judgments but rather, to determine what the risks are and how big they are. Risk assessments provide a basis from which the probabilities of occurrence of various, usually hazardous, events can be estimated. Based on the results of a risk assessment, decisions can be made concerning potential courses of action and the benefits to be gained from them. In making risk assessments, Lave (1987) points out that "risk analysts should not attempt to overstate or understate threats, but rather to give a best estimate and the range of uncertainty. Decision-makers can choose the proper amount of conservatism in setting the standard [for safety]" (p. 294). Overall, the usefulness of risk assessment depends on the magnitude of the uncertainties that are inherent in the information on which the assessment is based.

RISK AND UNCERTAINTY

"Risk" refers to the probability that given event, usually a negative one, will occur. "Uncertainty" refers to the margin of error in estimating the occurrence of the event. Risk and uncertainty are related to each other because both are influenced by the quality of relevant information that is available. As more and better information becomes available, the levels of risk and uncertainty can be more precisely set.

In assessing the risk of a particular event, it is important to determine whether the available information on which the assessment will be based was obtained from populations that share similar characteristics with the population for which the assessment is being made and whether there have been adequate controls for confounding variables. Lave (1987) notes that such controls are frequently not present; studies that serve as the basis for risk assessments often have the problems of "too few subjects for confident conclusions, failure to control for important confounding factors, no data (or [few] data) on exposure, exposure levels many times greater than the standards being considered, inadequate diagnosis, [and] subjects lost to follow-up" (p. 292). Because the available information is often incomplete and imperfect, the level of uncertainty is often high.

RISK ESTIMATION BASED ON HISTORICAL DATA

Short of finding the perfect study to provide information for accurate risk assessments, one can obtain beneficial information by using historical data. For example, a variety of techniques have been employed in performing cesarean section deliveries, and the use of these techniques has been extensively documented. Thus a great deal of useful information is available on the risks associated with cesarean sections, on the alternative procedures available, and on the factors that influence the decisions made by patients and physicians. However, there are limitations to using this approach. Wilson and Crouch (1987) note that the historical data are helpful in making decisions only if there is a model available concerning the likelihood of future events being similar to events in the past. The data on cesarean section deliveries, for example, will provide information on what conditions existed in the past, but one must also know whether those conditions will exist in the future. The characteristics of the obstetric populations, the number of malpractice lawsuits, and the availability of alternative procedures are examples of significant variables that have the potential for change over time.

A second limitation to using the historical data approach is twofold. Wilson and Crouch (1987) point out that "we can only use the historical approach to estimating risks when the hazard has been present for some time and the risk is large enough to be directly measured" (p. 268). If there is no historical data base for a given event, it is sometimes possible to obtain information on several separate parts of the event and to put the information together in order to obtain a picture of the whole event. This approach describes what has been done in compiling some of the perinatal risk scales: Several conditions known to be associated with a particular outcome are included on a scale; the risk estimates or risk scores for the individual conditions are then added together in an effort to obtain an overall estimate of the risk involved in the outcome.

The summing of the risk estimates for individual conditions presents problems, however, because it is not known whether the conditions are additive or multiplicative, or reflect some other mathematical function. Lesinski (1975) notes that "appropriate statistical methods . . . could statistically differentiate the effects of such [conditions]. But there is no assurance that such a statistical differentiation is any better than one arrived at by good clinical judgment" (p. 601). However, the hope remains that appropriate statistical methods can be developed that would offer improvements over clinical judgment alone or that would supplement such judgment. New approaches to the screening of perinatal risks could be developed from different statistical views of the interactive nature of perinatal risks, using both historical data and data on large numbers of subjects to provide risk estimates for combinations of perinatal conditions. New approaches will also be possible with the advent of new technologies and with new knowledge concerning conditions that were hitherto unknown to produce negative perinatal outcomes.

As these new approaches are developed, there will frequently be instances when historical data are lacking or are insufficient for appropriate use. Further, some conditions that had not been considered to be associated with other conditions in influencing perinatal outcomes might be so considered in the future. For example, socioeconomic status (SES) has been found to influence perinatal outcomes, with low SES being related to a higher incidence of negative outcomes. However, SES has been only inconsistently included as a component in perinatal risk scales, perhaps because the conditions inherent in SES that have a negative impact on a pregnant woman are conditions that cannot be easily or quickly altered by therapeutic intervention, particularly in late pregnancy. However, as Lesinski (1975) notes, SES should be considered basic to preconceptional screening systems that are coupled with programs designed to moderate reproductive risks in the future.

> Applying screening techniques and preventive measures years before any conception occurs could pay rich dividends in improved reproductive performance. . . . Recent epidemiologic studies of low birthweight and congenital anomalies of the central nervous system demonstrate clearly the relation of socioeconomic status and maternal physique to pregnancy outcome and quality of progeny. (p. 601)

If antepartum screening is appropriate for early identification of perinatal risks, prepregnancy screening might be even more appropriate for some populations of women.

RISK VALUE VERSUS CERTAINTY OF INFORMATION

An important issue in risk assessment is the interaction of risk value (i.e., the number of negative outcomes that are expected) and certainty of the information on the relationship between a particular condition and a negative outcome. If a condition is known with a high level of certainty to produce a negative outcome, then the condition should have a high risk value. However, perception of risk values varies with the number of negative outcomes that occur. By way of illustration, Wilson and Crouch (1987) provide the example of vinyl chloride gas as an almost certain cause of angiosarcoma. However, because the number of workers exposed to vinyl chloride gas is small, and because the exposure of workers to this gas today is minimal, the number of cases of angiosarcoma is "no more than one cancer . . . in several years" (p. 269).

If risks were perceived only according to the certainty of the information on the relationship between condition and outcome, then, clearly, exposure to vinyl chloride gas would be perceived as having a high risk value. However, other factors also influence perceptions of risk, such as cultural or societal values, individual preferences, and assumptions rather than facts. These "other factors" play an important role in influencing the performance and interpretation of risk assessments. Indeed, they are important enough that they can raise or lower the perception of the risk value in disproportion to its actual value.

Certainty of information has additional meaning for perinatal risk assessments in which there are still many unknowns. Although the overall goal of perinatal risk assessments is to identify and remedy all risk conditions so that there is a certainty of a positive perinatal outcome, the goal obviously has been, and continues to be, difficult to attain. The number of conditions that are known to be certain producers of either positive or negative outcomes is small. Further, there are frequent instances when the expected outcomes are not attained. It is "unknown factors" that are believed to be responsible "for such surprises as perinatal death in obstetric circumstances that appeared to offer no or little risk or, in contrast, perfectly healthy babies from high-risk pregnancies" (Lesinski, 1975, p. 602).

Because it is difficult to improve the certainty of the information available on perinatal risks, it might be more fruitful to try to improve the certainty of only some types of positive outcomes (e.g., normal intellectual functioning or normal cognitive development). Such an approach would mean that other types of positive outcomes would be relegated to positions of lesser importance. Attempts to rank order various outcomes would no doubt produce serious discussions on the broad and narrow values of particular outcomes. However, an attempt to focus attention more closely on just what types of specific outcomes can be maximized might be useful and productive.

There should also be a greater focus on the known risks and benefits of the available perinatal interventions and treatment methods. Such a focus is an important aspect of determining the relationship between perinatal risk conditions and perinatal outcomes. Yet, the effects of neither general nor specific types of intervention and treatment are considered in risk assessments. The true magnitude of the effects of perinatal risks on outcomes cannot be determined without such information. Thus, though risk values in terms of numbers of negative outcomes are important, so are the certainties of risks that exist despite intervention and treatment.

A fuller picture of the ultimate effect of intervention and treatment on outcome would also provide the public with better information on the certainties and the unknowns regarding remediation of specific types of perinatal risks. Perinatal screening scales should also be developed to differentiate between conditions in pregnancy for which there are effective treatments and conditions for which there are no treatments. Health care professionals should screen for both types of conditions, since knowledge of untreatable conditions would be useful in preparing pregnant woman for potential negative outcomes and alternatives. Perhaps this approach would reduce the expectation that each pregnancy should and will have a positive outcome.

EXPRESSION OF RISKS

There are many ways in which risk can be expressed, including various statistical expressions and such expressions as impact on life expectancy, incidence of cancer and other diseases, and quality of life. Some expressions of risk are more difficult to understand, and/or less compelling for the general public, than others. For example, knowing that 300 people died in the crash of a commercial airplane seems to create more worry among air travelers than does the knowledge among automobile drivers that 45,600 people died in traffic accidents in 1985 (Koshland, 1987; Lave, 1987).

For perinatal risks, it is less clear that some expressions of risks are more significant or compelling than others, since prevention of birth defects seems to be a universally shared value.

However, Wilson and Schifrin (1980) argue that by creating a notion of "high risk" with regard to pregnancies, the expression of risk in pregnancy has taken on a different meaning: "Present day standards prescribe potentially optimal care for the high-risk patients and potentially less than optimal care for the low-risk patients. . . . In our view 'low-risk pregnancy' is not definable, except in retrospect" (p. 655). The labeling of a pregnancy as belonging to one class or another of pregnancy risk may be creating an illusion of certainty that is not based on reality. Because the expression of risk through such labeling has implications for the treatments and monitoring that are prescribed, it is critical that the interpretation of such expressions is correct.

CONCLUSION

The tasks remaining with regard to improving the certainty of perinatal risk assessments are formidable, yet the groundwork has been laid. Many conditions are known to be related to perinatal risks, and for most of these conditions, historical data are available. We must take a fresh approach to the development of screening scales for perinatal risk, integrating conditions that were hitherto unknown to influence outcomes, interactions among conditions, the role of treatments and interventions, and the specific characteristics of the obstetric population under study. It is essential that there be greater sophistication in the use of statistical models, in the design of research to provide data for determining the effectiveness of the screening, and in the use of follow-up studies of the infants produced by the pregnancies under study to determine the influence of perinatal risks beyond the perinatal period. The necessary research tools and populations are available for the next steps to be taken.

Glossary

WITH KAREN YAPLE

ABNORMAL FETAL POSITION. Any abnormality noted with regard to the position of the fetus in the uterus prior to the onset of labor. Examples include *transverse* or *breech positions* noted during the last weeks of pregnancy; turning (external version) may be attempted prior to labor to prevent abnormal presentation. Abnormal position may be secondary to the presence of some other condition, such as multiple pregnancy, placenta previa, uterine malformation, or myoma.

ABNORMAL PRESENTATION. An abnormal position of the fetus at the beginning of or during the descent through the birth canal. Generally, a head-first descent, called *vertex presentation,* is considered normal. Normal vertex presentations include *occiput anterior* (OA), *right occiput anterior* (ROA), and *left occiput anterior* (LOA). Any presentation that is not vertex—or, on some scales (e.g., the University of Colorado Neonatal Morbidity Risk Scale [UCNM] and the High-Risk Pregnancy Screening System [HRPSS], not occiput anterior—is scored as abnormal. If only "vertex" is noted on the record, the presentation is considered normal. Abnormal presentations include *persistent occiput posterior, breech, sinciput, face (mentoanterior), brow, transverse (scapuloanterior),* and *compound* presentations. On the UCNM and the HRPSS, further items may be scored in the case of an abnormal presentation, according to the type of delivery. For example, on the UCNM, if there is a breech presentation followed by vaginal delivery with the fetus remaining in the breech position, then both abnormal presentation and breech delivery position are scored.

ABORTIONS. Defined by Littman and Parmelee (1978) as the termination of pregnancy before the gestational age of 20 weeks or when fetal weight is less than 500 grams. Others define abortion as the termination of pregnancy prior to the point of viability (i.e., when gestational age is between 20 and 28 weeks or when fetal weight is less than 500 grams). *Miscarriages* or *spontaneous abortions* are considered to occur prior to 20 weeks' gestation or before fetal weight has reached 500 grams. If the medical record notes a miscarriage as having occurred otherwise, it is scored as fetal death, not as abortion. Between 20 and 28 weeks, medically induced abortions, including therapeutic, artificial, and induced abortions, and other surgical procedures to remove the products of conception are scored as abortions. *Displaced pregnancies,* including tubal, ectopic, and ampullar pregnancies as well as any other pregnancies involving extrauterine placement, are considered abortions. Surgical procedures to remove dermoid cysts, hydatid cysts, or molar pregnancies are not scored as abortions. *Habitual abortion* is defined as three or more consecutive spontaneous abortions.

ACCIDENTS/SURGERY. Traumatic events such as accidents, abdominal surgery, or undergoing general anesthesia are scored on some scales (e.g., the UCNM). Accidents (e.g., automobile accidents or falls) noted in the medical record are scored. Surgery during pregnancy is scored if it is abdominal and/or if general anesthesia is used.

ACUTE SPECIFIC INFECTIONS. Specified infections occurring during pregnancy are scored as follows: *Urinary tract infections* (UTIs) that occur during pregnancy, respond to treatment, and do not recur later in the pregnancy are considered acute. On Maternal–Child Health Care Index (MCHCI), a history of frequent or chronic UTIs with a recurrence of infection during pregnancy is scored as chronic; the recurrence during pregnancy is not scored as acute. On this scale, UTIs include infections of the urethra *(urethritis),* bladder *(cystitis),* and kidneys *(pyelitis,* but excluding kidney disease). On the HRPSS, cystitis or *pyelonephritis* that occurs during pregnancy is scored as acute, regardless of the history of prior infection, on this scale "cystitis" refers to cystitis, bladder infection, or UTI. *Syphilis* during pregnancy is scored on some scales according to whether or not it is treated, or whether or not it is present at term.

ACUTE SYSTEMIC ILLNESSES. A variety of acute systemic conditions that can arise during pregnancy. On the HRPSS, the following conditions are scored as described: *Positive serology* refers to the pathological result of a test of the blood or other serum; infection or disease may be indicated by the test, but the individual may be asymptomatic.

Flu syndrome would be considered severe if there were excessive vomiting or dehydration. *Viral diseases* would include herpes virus infection, rubella, chicken pox, and mumps. *Fever* (temperature over 101°F) is scored as it is noted, regardless of the type of disease or infection. On the MCHCI, acute systemic conditions are scored according to whether the impact on the woman or the potential risk to the fetus is mild or serious; for example, severe flu syndrome or a viral disease such as rubella would be scored as a serious acute systemic illness.

AMNIOCENTESIS. Scored as noted in the medical record.

AMNIONITIS. Inflammation of the amnion. Amnionitis is also called *amniotitis.* Diagnosis may be confirmed by elevated maternal temperature or by bacteria in the amniotic fluid (which is suggested by the presence of nitrazine).

ANEMIA. Hemoglobin in the blood below normal range for the neonate or for the mother during pregnancy. On most scales, a mother's hemoglobin level of less than 9 grams per 100 milliliters of blood is considered to indicate severe anemia, and a level of 9–11 grams per 100 milliliters, mild anemia. The level of hemoglobin necessary for scoring anemia varies from scale to scale.

APGAR SCORE. The Apgar scoring system is used to rate the infant's overall condition at 1 minute and at 5 minutes after birth. Five areas—heart rate, respiratory effort, muscle tone, reflex irritability, and color—are rated on a scale of 0 to 2 and then summed. A score of 10 represents optimality. Scores below 7 or 8 represent below-optimum conditions, and scores below 5 represent greater risk.

APNEA. Brief episodes when breathing stops.

BLEEDING IN PREGNANCY. On most scales, vaginal bleeding at any time during pregnancy is scored. On the Obstetrical Complications Scale (OCS), "bleeding here may cover the spectrum from minimal spotting to hemorrhage and may occur at any time." On the HRPSS, minor bleeding is scored as *vaginal spotting,* and more serious bleeding, such as bleeding secondary to a placental problem, is scored according to the principal diagnosis. On the Labor Index (LI), bleeding is scored, first, according to severity; if it is not scored as severe, it is scored according to when, during the pregnancy, it occurs. Bleeding with pain or hypotension, and bleeding for which the mother is hospitalized, are scored according to whether the bleeding occurred before 20 weeks' gestation or after.

BLOOD TYPE PROBLEMS (maternal). Problems of *Rh sensitization* in the mother. On the HRPSS, one of two prenatal risk factors may be scored hierarchically: fetal exchange transfusion for Rh factor during a prior pregnancy or Rh sensitization. *Sensitization* is indicated by the presence of Rh antibodies (anti-Rh agglutinin) in the mother's blood or by prior fetal or infant Rh problems. Sensitization may be the result of the mother's failure to receive Rhogam at 28 weeks' gestation or at the termination of pregnancy for each pregnancy. The problem of Rh sensitization is also scored on the MCHCI and on the LI.

BLOOD TYPE PROBLEMS (infant). In the neonate, *Rh problems* or *ABO incompatibility* are specifically scored on the UCNM and the OCS, whereas the resulting symptoms or complications of hematologic problems are scored on the HRPSS and the Postnatal Complications Scale (PNCS). Generally, Rh problems are less common and more severe than problems related to ABO incompatibility. The following terms would most likely describe Rh problems, but they can also be used to describe the effects of ABO incompatibility: *exchange transfusion, erythroblastosis fetalis, hemolytic jaundice/anemia/disease of the newborn,* or *fetal hydrops. Icterus gravis neonatorum* is usually due to Rh problems. Icterus neonatorum refers to a mild, self-limiting case of hemolytic jaundice of the newborn, which would be more likely to be due to ABO incompatibility. There are other forms of icterus that would not be scored here, and alone, the term means jaundice. *Icterus, jaundice,* or *hyperbilirubinemia* are symptomatic of blood type problems, but they are insufficient indicators. As such, ABO incompatibility is scored if noted in the medical record or if diagnosed by a positive Coombs' test. Any Rh problems are scored if noted in the record. Related terms are scored as Rh problems if the mother's blood type is Rh negative and sensitization is indicated.

CEPHALOPELVIC DISPROPORTION (CPD). In cases of CPD, the fetal head is too large for the pelvic outlet of the mother, and vaginal delivery is impeded. The HRPSS distinguishes between small pelvis and clinical small pelvis: *Small pelvis* is scored according to the physician's assessment of an inadequate pelvic outlet early in the pregnancy, whereas *clinical small pelvis* is scored on the basis of the size of the pelvic outlet relative to the fetal head at delivery. In the case of a small pelvis, clinical small pelvis would not also be scored unless vaginal delivery was attempted and CPD became evident. Typically, CPD or clinical small pelvis refers to a pelvis of normal size that is functionally inadequate. In some cases of CPD, it may be necessary to deliver the infant vaginally. Further complications of delivery, such as cesarean section or forceps delivery, are scored in addition to CPD as they occur.

CESAREAN SECTION. Scored as noted in the medical record. May be described as *cervical, classical, extraperitoneal, cesarotomy,* or *cesarean hysterectomy.* A *transverse incision* may be noted and should be distinguished from a transverse presentation of the fetus. To be scored as a *planned cesarean section,* the record must indicate planning in advance of labor. Planning should not be assumed in the case of a repeat cesarean, since having had a prior cesarean no longer necessitates that subsequent deliveries be by cesarean.

CHRONIC HYPERTENSION/RENAL DISEASE. *Chronic hypertension,* or *hyperpiesis,* refers to chronic high blood pressure with an onset prior to the current pregnancy. It is considered mild when treated by diet, exercise, and observation, and severe when treated by medication or when it occurs with kidney damage or disease. Typically, *kidney* or *renal disease* excludes mild UTIs involving the pelvis or the kidneys (e.g., pyelitis, pyelocystitis, and pyelonephritis). On the HRPSS, renal disease is scored according to its severity, not its type. On that scale, *severe pyelonephritis* requiring hospitalization, for example, would be scored as moderate to severe renal disease. Nephritis, nephrosis, and nephropathy are scored as nephritis on the MCHCI, but as moderate to severe renal disease on the HRPSS. On the HRPSS, nephritis, if present, is scored in addition to chronic hupertension, whereas on the MCHCI, only nephritis would be scored.

CHRONIC SYSTEMIC ILLNESSES/CHRONIC DISEASES AND INFECTIONS. *Systemic illnesses* are illnesses that affect the whole body rather than one part. *Chronic diseses* are any diseases that occur repeatedly or are of long duration. To be scored as chronic on some scales, the disease must be present during the current pregnancy, regardless of the efficacy of treatment. Chronic pain due to injury, and psychological disorders, such a bipolar affective disorder or schizophrenia, that have biological bases, would not be scored here as either chronic or systemic. Psychosomatic disorders would be included if chronic and/or systemic. On the MCHCI, any illness scored according to its specific diagnosis is excluded from the definition of systemic. On this scale, a mother's chronic systemic illness is scored as debilitating or nondebilitating, according to how she experiences the effects of the illness. A debilitating illness is one that interferes with the mother's normal daily function or that causes permanent degenerating or disabling alteration of tissue or function. Normal daily function is considered to be compromised if the mother is unable to work or unable to care for herself without assistance prior to her pregnancy. Some examples of chronic debilitating systemic illnesses include acquired immune deficiency syndrome, systemic lupus erythematosus, multiple sclerosis, and muscular dystrophy. Some examples of nondebilitating chronic systemic diseses include chronic viral infections such as herpes zoster (shingles) and any chronic systemic diseses that are asymptomatic, responsive to treatment, or otherwise nondebilitating to the mother.

CHRONIC URINARY TRACT INFECTIONS (UTIs). Infections of the urethra, bladder, and kidneys (excluding kidney disease), such as urethritis, cystitis, and pyelitis, respectively. To be scored as chronic on the MCHCI, any UTI must have occurred at least twice prior to and/or during the current pregnancy, or the UTI must have been of long duration, beginning prior to and continuing into the pregnancy. A UTI that occurs only once and only during pregnancy is scored as acute on the MCHCI. On the HRPSS, recurring or persistent cystitis, bladder infection, or UTI prior to pregnancy is scored as history of cystitis. A history of pyelitis refers to one occurrence, prior to pregnancy, of pyelitis, pyelocystitis, pyelonephritis, or some other kidney infection not considered to be kidney disease.

CONTRACTED PELVIS. The condition in which one or more of the principal diameters of the pelvic outlet are reduced to the degree that parturition is impeded. A pelvis that is too small overall may be described as justo minor, dwarf, reduced, infantile, juvenile, nanous, or small. Additionally, certain shapes are likely to be considered contracted (i.e., beaked, flat, or funnel shaped.) Although there are many terms that could describe the borderline or contracted pelvis, the item is usually scored as *borderline* or *contracted* only if so described on the medical record. A small pelvis, described by any synonym, would be scored as "contracted" on the MCHCI and as "small" on the HRPSS.

CORD PROBLEMS. Scored as noted on the medical record. *Nuchal* refers to the umbilical cord's being wrapped around the neck. A *knotted cord* may be described as having a true knot. *Cord prolapse* refers to premature delivery of the cord (e.g., a section may be delivered before the shoulders are delivered). All of these examples are problematic because compression of the cord compromises the baby's blood and oxygen supply. If the cord is described as *compressed,* examine the record for additional information, to determine if it should be scored here.

DAMAGED INFANT. An infant who acquires an abnormality during labor and delivery or an abnormality that is due to some perinatal trauma. The abnormality is scored as either neurological or physical, the latter by the exclusion of not being neurological. Neurological damage would not be assumed from the presence of seizures.

DIABETES. This item is scored if noted in the medical history of the mother or during the gestational period for the current pregnancy. *Type I, Class A-II,* or *overt diabetes* refers to insulin-dependent diabetes of early onset, sometimes called *juvenile diabetes; brittle diabetes* would be scored in this category. *Type II* or *Class A-I diabetes* is less severe; *gestational diabetes* or *prediabetes* would be scored in this category. Treatment of diabetes in this second category is either by diet or by drugs such as Dimelor, Orinase, or Diabinese. *Maternal diabetes* is scored here as diabetes of any type. *Undetected diabetes* is considered here to be diabetes of any type that affects the mother and is untreated for more than one trimester of the pregnancy.

DRUGS/MEDICATION DURING PREGNANCY. Typically refers to prescription drugs, although drug abuse is also included on some scales. On the Rochester Research Obstetrical Scale (RROS), prescription drugs used on a chronic basis and continued during the current pregnancy are scored as *chronic medication.* On the OCS, prescription "drugs used on an acute basis during pregnancy" are scored, but vitamins, iron, and those drugs involved in drug abuse are excluded. However, there is a separate item for *drug abuse,* defined as "all drugs used illegally. . . . This may include approved medications used in an abusive fashion [tranquilizers, sleeping pills, pain medication] . . . alcohol, LSD, marijuana, etc." *Smoking* is included as drug abuse on the OCS. On the HRPSS *excessive use of drugs* is scored for illegal drug use or prescription or alcohol abuse. Heavy smoking is scored as a separate item on this scale. Moderate, nonabusive use of alcohol is also scored specifically on the HRPSS.

DRUGS IN LABOR. Of importance for scoring purposes are the types and amounts of drugs. On the OCS, any drugs administered during labor and delivery are scored, excluding local perineal anesthetics. On other scales, only specific types and/or dosages of drugs are scored. For example, magnesium sulfate ($MgSO_4$) is usually administered for toxemia; it is scored on the HRPSS if the total dosage exceeds 25 grams. *Analgesics* are scored according to the total dosage of all types. On the HRPSS, *Demerol* (meperidine hydrochloride) in excess of 300 milligrams is scored specifically. Some other examples of analgesics include *morphine, Sublimaze, Nisintel, Darvon,* and *Tylenol II* (with codine). Sedatives–hypnotics, tranquilizers, and drugs used to potentiate the effects of analgesics or anesthesia (e.g., *Seconal, Valium* [diazepam], *Phenergan, Largon, Vistaril*) would be scored in the general category of *labor and delivery drugs.* These types of drugs would not be scored in the specific categories for analgesia or anesthesia. *Anesthesia* is usually described in the medical record by the terms used for scoring. Typically, regional and general types of anesthesia are scored whereas local anesthesia is not. Types of regional anesthesia include *caudal, epidural, paracervical, pudendal, saddle,* and *spinal.* On the RROS, regional anesthesia must have been given in a higher total dosage than local or pudendal in order to be scored. On the HRPSS, general anesthesia is the only type of anesthesia that is scored.

DYSFUNCTIONS OF LABOR. *Primary dysfunctional labor* refers to primary uterine inertia, or a situation where the onset of labor is indicated by the rupture of membranes or some cervical dilation, up to 3–4 centimeters, but contractions are essentially absent or inefficient such that the progression of labor is less than 1–1.5 centimeters' per hour. *Prolonged latent stage* is similar to primary dysfunctional labor, except that the latent stage is pontaneously followed by active labor. Primary dysfunctional labor or sprolonged latent stage are scored only as noted. *Secondary arrest of dilation* refers to failure to progress after 5 centimeters' dilation. The phrase "failure to progress" (FTP) may be used in the medical record to describe either primary dysfunctional labor or a secondary arrest of dilation. However, FTP alone is insufficient for scoring here, and information about the progress of labor or the dilation of the cervix is needed for differentially scoring FTP in either of these categories.

EMOTIONAL PROBLEM. Any emotional problem for which the mother has been hospitalized or has received medication is scored on the HRPSS. Excessive anxiety, acute grief reaction, or any clinically diagnosed psychological disorder that is present during the current pregnancy is also scored.

ENDOCRINE DISORDERS. Disorders of the thyroid, parathyroid, adrenals, pituitary, pancreas, or ovaries. Diabetes (pancreas), sterility due to ovarian dysfunction, and ovarian cysts are scored elsewhere.

Definite *adrenal* or *pituitary problems* include Addison disease, Cushing disease or syndrome, primary aldosteronism, and growth disorders. *Thyroid problems* or *diseases* include hypoparathyroidism and hyperparathyroidism or osteitis fibrosa cystica generalisata. *Endocrine ablation* (the surgical removal of all or part of any endocrine gland) is scored, except for kidney removal, which is scored only if removal of the adrenal gland is noted. *Ovariectomy* (the surgical removal of an ovary for any reason) would be scored, although removal of an ovarian cyst or ovarian resection would not be scored.

ENDOCRINE DISORDERS (other). Terms describing recurrent menstrual dysfunction include, for example, *amenorrhea, polyhypomenorrhea,* or *polymenorrhea.* Dysmenorrhea is not scored. *Infertility* is scored if noted in the medical record, with one exception: If it is specifically noted to be secondary to scarring of the fallopian tubes or to have been caused by infection (i.e., gonorrhea, pelvic inflammatory disease), it is not considered an endocrine dysfunction and thus is not scored. On the OCS, *prolonged unwanted sterility* refers to those situations where conception has been unsuccessful for more than 2 years.

EPILEPSY. Scored if the patient is noted to have epilepsy or repeated seizures.

FAMILY HISTORY OF DIABETES. The presence of diabetes in any first- or second-degree maternal relatives.

FETAL ACIDOSIS. May result from hypoxic conditions during labor and is symptomatic of fetal distress. It is scored according to a fetal or cord blood pH level of less than 7.25.

FETAL OR CONGENITAL ANOMALY (prior infants). The intrauterine development of an organ or structure that is abnormal in form, structure, or position. A synonym is *birth defect.*

FETAL DEATH/STILLBIRTH. Death of the fetus after 32 weeks' gestation, or after the fetus has reached a weight greater than 500 grams, such that the fetus dies in the uterus and must be removed or is dead at birth.

FETAL DISTRESS. Although a number of items may indicate fetal distress, it is scored on the UCNM only as noted in the medical record. On other scales, the specific symptoms of fetal distress, such as the presence of meconium, fetal heart rate abnormalities, and fetal acidosis, are scored as noted in the medical record.

FETAL HEART RATE (abnormalities). Any heart rate acceleration—for example, *tachycardia* (mild, if 151 to 180 beats per minute; moderate, if 181 to 200 beats per minute; severe, if over 200 beats per minute)—or deceleration—for example, *bradycardia* (mild, if 100 to 109 beats per minute; moderate, if 80 to 90 beats per minute; severe, if less than 80 beats per minute)— is noted. On the LI, the OCS, and the RROS, the length of time is not considered. However, the HRPSS specifies that high or low heart rate must occur for more than 30 minutes to be scored.

FORCEPS. The use of forceps is scored here. *Outlet forceps* may be low, mid, or high; *operative forceps* and *vacuum extraction* would be scored as noted or if used in the attempt to turn a malpresenting fetus. On the HRPSS, vacuum extraction and operative forceps are scored in the same category. On the UCNM, the use of forceps or vacuum extraction is scored as a delivery complication.

GENERATIVE TRACT DISORDERS. *Uterine malformation* refers to abnormal structural congenital formations, such as a septum dividing the uterus. Other terms include unicornis, bicornis, biforis, bilocularis, bipartite, cordiformis, didelphys, or double uterus. Displacements of the uterus, such as a tipped or prolapsed uterus, are not scored. *Myomas* are uterine tumors, which also may be referred as fibroids or fibromata. *Endometriosis* involves extrauterine displacement of the lining of the uterus (endometrium); it is scored only if noted. *Pelvic inflammatory disease* may be associated with endometriosis, but it is scored as an acute or chronic disease, not as a generative tract disorder. *Incompetent cervix* is scored as noted, as are ovarian masses, cysts, or tumors. Incompetent cervix may be assumed if cerclage has been performed. *Abnormal cervical cytology* refers to abnormal cell structure, which may be noted by an abnormal (Class II or above) Pap (Papanicalaou) test. On the MCHCI, incompetent cervix is categorized with known cervical anomalies, which include abnormal cytology, benign cervical cysts, and structural abnormalities such as those resulting from previous tears, lacerations, cauterization, or cryotherapy.

GESTATIONAL AGE. May be determined by the date of the mother's last menstrual period or by maturity ratings such as the Dubowitz score. Optimal gestational age is between 38 and 42 weeks.

HEART DISEASE. Any pathological condition of the heart—for example, endocarditis, myocarditis, pericarditis, coronary artery occlusion, valve problems, congenital malformations, and arrhythmia. The classification system considers the irregularity of the heart beat. Irregularities that can be detected only by electrocardiogram are scored as *Class I.* Other problems are scored according to the severity indicated, with *Class II* usually considered a mild disorder and *Class III* or *Class IV* the most severe. If there is a history of heart failure, heart attack, cardiac arrest, myocardial infarction, or congestive heart failure regardless of any heart disease, it is scored alone on some scales (eg., the MCHCI) and as severe heart disease on other scales (e.g., the HRPSS). *Murmurs* are scored on most scales as Class I heart disease.

HYDRAMNIOS OR OLIGOHYDRAMNIOS. *Hydramnios* refers to an excess of liquor amnii, which may be due to multiple pregnancy or to an abnormality of the fetus. Specifically, it is defined as an amount of amniotic fluid greater than 2,500 milliliters at the intrapartum period. *Polyhydramnios* also refers to the presence of an excessive amount of amniotic fluid. *Oligohydramnios,* on the other hand, refers to an abnormally small amount of amniotic fluid. On the HRPSS, polyhydramnios is scored if the excess of amniotic fluid is noted during the prenatal period; hydramnios is scored if the excess is noted during the intrapartum period. During the intrapartum period, either oligohydramnios or hydramnios increases the possiblity of fetal malpresentation.

HYPEREMESIS. Excessive vomiting. Only vomiting that is excessive enough to require hospitalization is scored.

INDUCTION/PITOCIN. Labor may be induced by stripping the membranes (amniotomy) or by using oxytocins, such as Pitocin. Either procedure may be used to expedite labor, so induction must be noted in the medical record in order to be scored. Administration of oxytocins prior to delivery without induction being noted in the record, or administration during the first or second stage of labor, would be scored as *Pitocin augmentation.* Distinctions between induction and augmentation may be made by noting the temporal sequence of the onset of labor and the administration of Pitocin. *Induction* for any medical reason would be scored as a medical induction. Induction for other than a medical reason would be scored as an elective induction.

INFANT CENTRAL NERVOUS SYSTEM DEPRESSION. Decreased function of the central nervous system which is characterized by symptoms ranging from floppiness to coma, including poor muscle tone, reflex abnormalities, lack of spontaneous respiration, and hypothermia.

INFANT CONVULSION. Any clonic, tonic, or repetitive activity of a tremulous nature that the medical staff believed to be a seizure. This item is scored as noted in the medical record by the physician.

INFANT DYSMATURITY. Abnormally small size of the infant relative to what would be expected according to the gestational age.

INFANT FAILURE TO GAIN WEIGHT. Wasting due to malabsorption, metabolic disorder, or vitamin deficiencies.

INFANT FEEDING PROBLEMS. Difficulties that inhibit feeding, such as disinterest, poor suck, or emesis. This item is intended to be an assessment of the infant's general state of health around the time of birth. On the PNCS, feeding within 48 hours of birth is considered optimal. If feedings are begun normally but are discontinued later, then the item is still scored optimally.

INFANT HEMORRHAGIC PROBLEMS. Specific conditions include hemorrhagic diathesis and hemorrhagic disease of the newborn. Administration of vitamin K can correct the conditions.

INFANT HYPERBILIRUBINEMIA. Generally defined as a bilirubin level greater than 14 milligrams percent (per 100 milliliters), although other levels are also used.

INFANT INFECTION (positive or suspected). Any infectious illness affecting any part of the infant's body. The site may be as superficial as the skin or as deep seated as sepsis. Similarly, the degree of infection may range from very mild to very serious. The term *suspected* means that the infection need not be proven by culture techniques but merely must be suspected by the physician. Thus treatment of suspected sepsis would be scored affirmatively.

INFANT METABOLIC DISTURBANCES. Disturbances that are usually diagnosed by examinations of bodily fluids. Inborn errors of metabolism are also covered under this item. The most common disturbances are hypoglycemia; hypocalcemia; hypomagnesemia or hypermagnesemia; hypoparathyroidism; failure to gain weight; and jitteriness or hyperactivity with specific causes.

INFANT NONINFECTIOUS ILLNESS OR ANOMALY. Any

structural or functional abnormality. It specifically excludes any type of infection. Minor skin anomalies are not typically included. Some examples included on the PCS are cerebral hemorrhage, hydrocephalus, hypospadias, ambiguous genitalia, umbilical hernia, intestinal obstruction, patent ductus arteriosus, coronary heart disease, and shock.

INFANT PERSISTENT CYANOSIS. *Cyanosis* is blue color due to lack of oxygen and excess of carbon dioxide in the blood. *Persistent cyanosis* refers to the continuation of this condition more than 1 hour postnatally.

INFANT RESPIRATORY DISTRESS. The occurrence of respiratory distress in any form would elicit a positive response to this item. *Distress* is defined as one or more of the following: (1) grunting, (2) retractions, (3) respiratory rate greater than 60 breaths per minute, and (4) nasal flaring. The distress must be present for more than an hour to be scored on the OCS.

INFANT SURGERY. Surgery refers to (1) any procedure performed under general anesthesia by a surgeon (including all endoscopic techniques) and (2) any procedure requiring an incision through the skin. Certain procedures, however, are not typically included here, such as spinal taps, circumcisions, cutdowns, subdural taps, ventricular taps, and other nonanesthetic radiologic studies.

INFANT TEMPERATURE DISTURBANCE. Any temperature outside the range of 36–37.5°C. Because hypothermic temperatures are commonly found in infants in the delivery room after birth, a positive response refers only to those situations arising at least 1 hour postnatally.

INFANT VENTILATORY ASSISTANCE. This item is intended to define further complications of *infant respiratory distress*. It includes the use of any of the following methods in the support of respiration: (1) intermittent positive pressure breathing, (2) continuous positive-pressure breathing, (3) continuous positive airway pressure, or (4) negative chest wall pressure. These methods may be administered by mask or by endotracheal intubation. Items pertaining to *resuscitation at birth* usually are referring to administration of any of the methods listed here.

LABOR COMPLICATIONS. A number of specific items are

scored in this category, including the following: induction of labor, administration of Pitocin or other oxytocins, contracted pelvis, uterine inertia, primary dysfunctional labor, and maternal shock.

LENGTH OF LABOR. Record the times for Stage I and Stage II labor. The length of time for each stage is used as the basis for the risk score as noted on each scale. Even if delivery is by cesarean section, the length of time for each stage, if available, can be scored.

MARITAL STATUS. The mother's marital status at delivery, scored as married or single. "Married" includes legally married, and married but separated. "Single" includes divorced, widowed, and unmarried cohabitation.

MATERNAL AGE. The mother's age at delivery.

MECONIUM. The presence of meconium stool in the amniotic fluid is a symptom of fetal distress during labor or delivery and places the infant at risk for *meconium aspiration syndrome*. The *amniotic fluid* is usually assessed for meconium at the time or rupture of the membranes. The fluid may be described as clear, indicating no meconium; as cloudy, turbid, or bloody; or according to the color or viscosity of the discharge. Meconium also may appear later in labor; appearance at any time should be scored. On scales that rate the amniotic fluid, turbid, light, or thin meconium indicates lower risk, whereas gross, bloody, heavy, dark, or thick meconium indicates higher risk.

MULTIPLE PREGNANCY. Scored as noted in the medical record. Pregnancies involving twins usually are not distinguished from other multiple pregnancies. On the HRPSS, this item is scored as a prenatal risk factor and as an intrapartum risk factor. Live multiple birth, also on this scale, is scored as a neonatal risk factor.

NEONATAL DEATH. Death of an infant that occurs at birth or up to 6 weeks of age.

NUTRITION/WEIGHT. *Malnutrition* as scored here is not necessarily related to weight, although it may be more common when weight is either extremely low (under 100 pounds) or extremely high (over 200 pounds). Being nutritionally compromised or having any disease due to vitamin deficiency would be scored here as malnourished. *Obesity* is scored if the woman's weight is over 200 pounds at any time during pregnancy. *Inadequate diet* also is not necessarily related to weight; it refers to a diet low in calories but nutritionally complete. Low weight gain during pregnancy may indicate inadequate diet but should not be scored unless more specifically noted.

PARITY. The number of live infants born to a woman who were past 20 weeks' gestation and who weighed over 500 grams at birth. This definition, taken from Littman and Parmelee, excludes the current pregnancy and all abortions, fetal deaths, and stillbirths. Infants who died shortly after birth would be included in this definition. Others have defined parity as the number of pregnancies carried to the point of viability, regardless of the outcome. When this definition is used, fetal deaths and stillbirths are included.

PLACENTAL PROBLEM. On some scales (e.g., the RROS), any placental problem is scored. On other scales, specific problems are scored as they are noted. *Placenta previa* refers to implantation of the placenta in the lower uterine segment. It also can be described as placenta previa centralis, lateralis, marginalis, or partialis. Placenta previa presents to the mother and the fetus the risk of excessive blood loss and of premature cesarean delivery. *Abruptio placentae* (also ablatio placentae, abruption, or premature rupture of the placenta) refers to the separation, prior to the onset of labor, of a normally situated placenta. Abruptio placentae may be associated with toxemia, with such symptoms as hemorrhage and constant uterine contraction which is occasionally tetanic in nature. *Marginal separation* is an incomplete premature separation. *Antepartum hemorrhage* is hemorrhaging that occurs before the onset of labor. It may be caused by placenta previa, abruptio placentae, or marginal separation. *Placental infarction* refers to the presence of areas of necrosis in the placenta that are due to cessation of the blood supply. This is scored according to its diagnosis by the pathologist. If the infarcts present in a placenta are determined to be within the normal limit, placenta infarction is not scored.

POST-TERM. Typically refers to gestational age greater than 42 weeks.

PREMATURE OR LOW BIRTHWEIGHT INFANTS. *Premature infants* are those whose gestational age is less than 37 weeks. On the HRPSS and OCS, *low birthweight infants* are defined as those who weigh less than 2,500 grams at birth. On other scales (e.g., the UCNM and RROS), criteria for prematurity include low birthweight and/or gestational age. *Very low birthweight infants* are those who weigh less than 1,500 grams.

PREMATURE RUPTURE OF MEMBRANES. Membranes may rupture spontaneously *(SROM)* or may be artificially ruptured *(AROM)*. The time of rupture should be noted; it is compared to the time of delivery. *Premature rupture of membranes (PROM)* may occur prior to the onset of labor or may be associated with long labor. Sometimes the membranes are described as leaking and then resealing themselves prior to labor; only unsealed leaks or ruptures should be scored. The length of time between rupture and delivery that determines premature rupture varies across scales.

PRENATAL CARE. The number of visits made to an obstetrician during pregnancy as noted in the medical record and when (i.e., which trimester) the visits began. Sometimes the record is incomplete because of a change of doctors; this can be difficult to determine and should not be assumed.

PRIOR FETAL MALPRESENTATIONS. *Abnormal presentations* of fetuses that occurred during prior deliveries. These include breech, footling, transverse, compound, sinciput, face, brow, and shoulder presentations and any other presentations that were not vertex, occiput anterior, or occiput posterior.

PULMONARY DISEASE. Lung disease, for example, emphysema, chronic obstructive pulmonary disease, pneumonia, pleurisy, asthma, hay fever, and chronic bronchitis. On the HRPSS, *tuberculosis* or *purified protein derivative of tuberculin* over 10 millimeters (a positive test for tuberculosis) is scored separately. Diseases of the pulmonary artery or valve, such as *pulmonary stenosis,* are scored as heart disease rather than as pulmonary disease.

RACE. The race or ethnicity of the mother, scored as white or nonwhite. White means Caucasion; nonwhite includes black, Native American, Indian, Asian, Latin, and others.

RESPIRATORY DISTRESS SYNDROME (RDS). Formerly called *hyaline membrane disease,* RDS is a condition in which the lungs are not mature enough to produce pulmonary surfactant. Symptoms include delayed onset of respiration, cyanosis, floppiness, heart failure, and symptoms of respiratory distress (grunting, retractions, increased respiratory rate, and nasal flaring).

SEPSIS. Infection that is typically accompanied by fever and detected by the presence of microorganisms in the bloodstream. Such infection may be localized or widespread. On scales of optimality, any type of infection affecting any part of the body is scored. Infections not proven by culture techniques, but which are suspected and treated prophylactically by the physician, are also scored.

SHOULDER DYSTOCIA. Difficulty in the delivery of an infant's shoulders; associated with trauma to the infant's shoulders or arms during delivery. It is scored only as noted in the medical record.

TIME SINCE LAST PREGNANCY. The time between the termination of a woman's last pregnancy and the current delivery. Termination of the prior pregnancy is noted regardless of the outcome, including abortion, displaced pregnancy, or fetal death. On the OCS, this item is scored as a risk factor if the time interval is less than 12 months.

TOXEMIA AND RELATED SYMPTOMS. *Toxemia* is characterized by high blood pressure, protein in the urine, edema, and abnormal reflexes. It also is referred to as *pre-eclampsia* and may progress to *eclampsia*. The hallmarks of eclampsia are coma and convulsive seizures. On the HRPSS, distinctions are made in scoring according to when the toxemia occurred. Toxemia may occur between the 20th week of pregnancy and the end of the 1st week postpartum. History of toxemia (or of eclampsia) is scored if toxemia (or eclampsia) was a complication of a prior pregnancy. Toxemia during the current pregnancy is scored according to its presence during the prenatal and/or the intrapartum periods. On other scales, the occurrence of toxemia at any time during the current pregnancy is scored. On the HRPSS and the LI, toxemia (or pre-eclampsia) is also scored according to the severity indicated in the medical record. Toxemia (or pre-eclampsia) of any greater severity than mild is scored as severe. Eclampsia would be scored as severe toxemia, although toxemia is usually considered to be an attenuated form of eclampsia. Usually, treatment prevents the progression of symptoms to eclampsia. Two symptoms, high blood pressure and protein in the urine, are scored as they occur alone or as noted in the context of toxemia, on the OCS. Single occurrences of hypertension (blood pressure greater than 140/90) and of albuminuria (a lab value greater than 2+ for protein in the urine) are scored on this scale. Treatment for toxemia essentially involves control of high blood pressure and frequent monitoring of symptoms. High blood pressure may be treated with Apresoline or Hydralyn, trade names for hydralazine hydrochloride. Magnesium sulfate (Epsom salt, $MgSO_4$) may be administered intravenously. If the symptoms of toxemia cannot be controlled, or if the length of gestation of the fetus is greater than 37 weeks, the pregnancy may be terminated by inducing labor or by cesarean section.

UTERINE RUPTURE. Scores as noted in the medical record. Attempting vaginal birth after cesarean (VBAC) is associated with risk of uterine rupture.

UTERINE TETANY. Prolonged or excessive uterine contractions. Uterine tetany may cause a premature rupture or separation of the placenta and decreased uteroplacental blood flow.

References

Akhtar, J., & Sehgal, N. N. (1980). Prognostic value of a prepartum and intrapartum risk-scoring method. *Southern Medical Journal, 73,* 411–414.

Als, H. (1978). Assessing an assessment: Conceptual considerations, methodological issues, and a perspective on the future of the Neonatal Behavioral Assessment Scale. In A. Sameroff (Ed.), Organization and stability of newborn behaviors: A commentary on the Brazelton Neonatal Behavioral Assessment Scale (pp. 14–28). *Monographs of the Society for Research in Child Development, 43* (5–6, Serial No. 177).

Anderson, C. J. (1983). Enhancing responsiveness in mother–infant interaction. *Infant Behavior and Development, 6,* 361–368.

Apgar, V. (1953). A proposal for a new method of evaluation of the newborn infant. *Anesthesia and Analgesia: Current Research, 32,* 260–267.

Ascher, B. (1978). Maternal anxiety in pregnancy and fetal homeostasis. *Journal of Obstetric and Gynecological Nursing, 78,* 18–21.

Astbury, J. (1980). The crises of childbirth: Can information and childbirth education help? *Journal of Psychosomatic Research, 24,* 9–13.

Aubry, R., & Pennington, J. (1973). Identification and evaluation of high-risk pregnancy: The perinatal concept. *Clinical Obstetrics and Gynecology, 16,* 3–27.

Ballinger, C. (1982). Emotional disturbance during pregnancy and following delivery. *Psychosomatic Research, 26,* 629–634.

Barrera, M., & Balls, P. (1983). Assessing social support as a preventive resource: An illustrative study. *Prevention in Human Services, 2,* 59–74.

Baruffi, G., Strobino, D. M., & Dellinger, W., Jr. (1984). Definitions of high risk in pregnancy and evaluation of their predictive validity. *American Journal of Obstetrics and Gynecology, 148,* 781–786.

Batzofin, J. H., Fielding, W. L., & Friedman, E. A. (1984). Effect of vaginal bleeding in early pregnancy on outcome. *Obstetrics and Gynecology, 63,* 515–518.

Bayley, N. (1969). *Bayley Scales of Infant Development.* New York: Psychological Corporation.

Beck, A. T., Ward, C. H., Mendelson, M., Mock, J., & Erbaugh, J. (1961). An inventory for measuring depression. *Archives of General Psychiatry, 4,* 561–571.

Beck, N., Siegel, L., Davidson, W., Kormeier, J., Breitenstein, A., & Hall, D. (1980). Prediction of pregnancy outcome: Maternal preparation, anxiety and attitudinal sets. *Psychosomatic Research, 24,* 343–351.

Beckwith, L., & Cohen, S. (1980). Interactions of preterm infants with their caregivers and test performance at age 2. In T. Field, S. Goldberg, S. Stern, & A. Sostek (Eds.), *High-risk infants and children* (pp. 155–178). New York: Academic Press.

Beckwith, L., Cohen, S., & Parmelee, A. (1973, August). *Risk, sex, and situational influences in social interactions with premature infants.* Paper presented at the meeting of the American Psychological Association.

Bee, H., Barnard, K., Eyres, S., Gray, C., Hammond, M., Spietz, A., Snyder, C., & Clark, B. (1982). Prediction of IQ and language skills from perinatal status, child performance, family characteristics and mother–infant interaction. *Child Development, 53,* 1134–1156.

Berkowitz, G., & Kasl, S. (1983). The role of psychosocial factors in spontaneous preterm delivery. *Psychosomatic Research, 27,* 283–290.

Blau, A., Slaff, B., Easton, D., Welkowitz, J., & Cohen, J. (1963). The psychogenic etiology of premature births: A preliminary report. *Psychosomatic Medicine, 20,* 201–211.

Blau, A., Welkowitz, J., & Cohen, J. (1964). Maternal Attitude to Pregnancy Instrument. *Archives of General Psychiatry, 10,* 324–331.

Brazelton, T. B. (1973). *Neonatal Behavioral Assessment Scale, No. 50.* Philadelphia: J. B. Lippincott Co.

Broman, S., Nichols, P., & Kennedy, W. (1975). *Preschool IQ: Prenatal and early development correlates.* Hillsdale, NJ: Erlbaum.

Bukovsky, I., Herman, A., Sherman, D. Schreyer, P., Arieli, S., & Caspi, E. (1985). Perinatal outcome following physician's strike of 1983. *Israel Journal of Medical Science, 21,* 804–807.

Burstein, L., Kinch, R. A. H., & Stern, L. (1974). Anxiety, pregnancy, labor and the neonate. *American Journal of Obstetrics and Gynecology, 118,* 195.

Caldwell, B., & Bradley, R. (1978). *Manual of the Home Observation for Measurement of Environment.* Unpublished manuscript, University of Arkansas, Little Rock.

Campbell, S. K., & Wilhelm, I. J. (1985). Development from birth to 3 years of age of 15 children at high risk for central nervous system dysfunction. *Physical Therapy, 65,* 463–469.

Caputo, D., Goldstein, K., & Taub, H. (1981). Neonatal compromise and later psychological development: A 10-year longitudinal study. In S. Friedman & M. Sigman (Eds.), *Preterm birth and psychological development* (pp. 353–386). New York: Academic Press.

Carey, W., & McDevitt, S. (1978). Revision of the Infant Temperament Questionnaire. *Pediatrics, 61,* 735–739.

Carlson, D., & LaBarba, R. (1979). Maternal emotionality during pregnancy and reproductive outcome: A review of the literature. *International Journal of Behavior Development, 2,* 343–376.

Chalmers, B. (1981). A selective review of stress: Some cognitive approaches taken a step further. *Psychological Review, 1,* 325.

Chalmers, B. (1982). Psychological aspects of pregnancy: Some thoughts for the eighties. *Social Science Medicine, 16,* 323–331.

Chalmers, B. (1983). Psychosocial factors and obstetric complications. *Psychological Medicine, 13,* 333–339.

Chalmers, B. (1984). A conceptualization of psycho-social obstetric research. *Journal of Psychosomatic Obstetrics and Gynecology, 3,* 17–26.

Cohen, S., & Beckwith, L. (1979). Preterm infants' interaction with the caregiver in the first year of life and competence at age 2. *Child Development, 50,* 767–777.

Cohen, S. E., Parmelee, A. H., Sigman, M., & Beckwith, L. (1982). Neonatal risk factors in preterm infants. *Applied Research in Mental Retardation, 3,* 265–278.

Cohen, S. E., Sigman, M., Parmelee, A. H., & Beckwith, L. (1982). Perinatal risk and developmental outcome in pre-term infants. *Seminars in Perinatology—Review, 6,* 334–339.

Coopland, A. T., Peddle, L. J., Baskett, T. F., Rollwagen, R., Simpson, A., & Parker, E. (1977). A simplified antepartum high-risk pregnancy scoring form: Statistical analysis of 5459 cases. *Canadian Medical Association Journal, 116,* 999–1001.

Coplan, J. (1980). Spurious conclusions. *Pediatrics, 66,* 155–156.

Cox, L. C., Hack, M., & Metz, D. (1981). Brainstem-evoked response audiometry: Normative data from the preterm infant. *Audiology, 20,* 53–64.

Cox, L. C., Hack, M., & Metz, D. (1984). Auditory brain stem response abnormalities in the very low birthweight infant: Incidence and risk factors. *Ear and Hearing, 5,* 47–51.

Crandon, A. J. (1979). Maternal anxiety and neonatal well-being. *Journal of Psychosomatic Research, 23,* 113–115.

Davids, A., & DeVault, S. (1962). Maternal anxiety during pregnancy and childbirth abnormalities. *Psychosomatic Medicine, 24,* 464–470.

Davids, A., DeVault, S., & Talmadge, M. (1961). Anxiety, pregnancy and childbirth abnormalities. *Journal of Consulting and Clinical Psychology, 25,* 74–77.

Dixon, S. D., Tronick, E., Keefer, & Brazelton, T. B. (1982). Malnutrition: A closer look at an East African village. *Developmental Medicine and Child Neurology, 24,* 670–685.

Dohrenwend, B., Krasnoff, L., Askenasy, A., & Dohrenwend, B. (1978). Exemplification of a method for scaling live events: The PERI Life Events Scale. *Journal of Health and Social Behavior, 19,* 205.

Donahue, C., & Wan, T. (1975). Measuring obstetric risk of prematurity. *American Journal of Obstetrics and Gynecology, 116,* 911.

Edwards, K., & Jones, M. (1970). Personality changes related to pregnancy and obstetric complications. *Proceedings of the 78th Annual Convention of the American Psychological Association, 5,* 341–342.

Eskes, T. K., Timmer, H., Kollee, L. A., & Jongsma, H. W., (1985). The second twin. *European Journal of Obstetrics, Gynecology and Reproductive Biology, 19,* 159–166.

Feldstein, M., & Butler, N. (1965). Analysis of factors affecting perinatal mortality. *British Journal of Preventative Social Medicine, 19,* 128.

Ferreira, A. (1965). Emotional factors in the prenatal environment. *Journal of Nervous and Mental Disorders, 141,* 108–118.

Field, T., Hollock, N., Ting, G., Dempsey, J., Dabini, C., & Shuman, H. (1978). A first-year follow-up of high risk infants: Formulating a cumulative risk index. *Child Development, 49,* 119–131.

Field, T. M., Ignatoff, E., Stringer, S., Brennan, J., Greenberg, R., Widmayer, S., & Anderson, G. C. (1982). Nonnutritive sucking during tube feedings: Effects on preterm neonates in an intensive care unit. *Pediatrics, 70,* 381–384.

Field, T. M., Sandberg, D., Quetel, T. A., Garcia, R., & Rosario, M. (1985). Effects of ultrasound feedback on pregnancy anxiety, fetal activity, and neonatal outcome. *Obstetrics and Gynecology, 66,* 525–528.

Field, T. M., Widmayer, S., Stringer, S., & Ignatoff, E. (1980). Teenage, lower-class, black mothers and their preterm infants: An intervention and developmental follow up. *Child Development, 51,* 426–436.

Firestone, P., & Prabhu, A. N. (1983). Minor physical anomalies and obstetrical complications: Their relationship to hyperactive, psychoneurotic, and normal children and their families. *Journal of Abnormal Child Psychology, 11,* 207–216.

Forslund, M., & Bjerre, I. (1983). Neurological assessment of preterm infants at term conception age in comparison with normal full-term infants. *Early Human Development, 8,* 195–208.

Friedman, S. L. (1982). Complementing the success of medical intervention. *Seminars in Perinatology, 6,* 365–368.

Friedman, S. L., Jacobs, B. S., & Werthmann, M. W. (1982). Preterms of low medical risk: Spontaneous behaviors and soothability at expected date of birth. *Infant Behavior and Development, 5,* 3–10.

Funderburk, S. I., Guthrie, D., & Meldrum, D. (1980). Outcome of pregnancies complicated by early vaginal bleeding. *British Journal of Obstetrics and Gynecology, 87,* 100–105.

Georgas, J., Giakoumaki, E., Georgoulias, N., Koumandakis, E., & Kaskarelis, D. (1984). Psychosocial stress and its relation to obstetrical complications. *Psychotherapy and Psychosomatics, 41,* 200–206.

Goldstein, K., Caputo, D., & Taub, H. (1976). The effects of prenatal and perinatal complications on development at one year of age. *Child Development, 47,* 613–621.

Goodwin, J. W., Dunne, J. T., & Thomas, B. W. (1969). Antepartum identification of the fetus at risk. *Canadian Medical Association Journal, 101,* 57–65.

Gorsuch, R. L., & Key, M. K. (1974). Abnormalities of pregnancy as a function of anxiety and life stress. *Psychosomatic Medicine, 36,* 352–367.

Green, W. H. (1984). A comparison of schizophrenic and autistic children. *Journal of the American Academy of Child Psychiatry, 23,* 399–409.

Grimm, E. (1967). Psychological and social factors in pregnancy, delivery and outcome. In S. A. Richardson & A. F. Guttmacher (Eds.), *Childbearing: Its social and psychological aspects* (pp. 520–527). Baltimore, MD: Williams & Wilkins.

Gross, T., Sokol, R. J., & King, K. C. (1980). Obesity in pregnancy: Risks and outcome. *Obstetrics and Gynecology, 56,* 446–450.

Gunter, L. (1963). Psychopathology and stress in the life experience of mothers of premature infants. *American Journal of Obstetrics and Gynecology, 86,* 333–340.

Halliday, H. L., Jones, P. K., & Jones, S. L. (1980). Method of screening obstetric patients to prevent reproductive wastage. *Obstetrics and Gynecology, 55,* 656–661.

Hobel, C. (1975). Recognition of the high risk pregnant woman. In W. Spellacy (Ed.), *Proceedings of the Symposium on the High Risk Pregnancy, March 1975.* Baltimore: University Park Press.

Hobel, C. J. (1978). Risk assessment in perinatal medicine. *Clinical Obstetrics and Gynecology, 21,* 287–295.

Hobel, C. J. (1980). Better perinatal health. *Lancet, 1,* 31–33.

Hobel, C. J., Hyvarinen, M. A., Okada, D. M. & Oh, W. (1973). Prenatal and intrapartum high-risk screening: I. Prediction of the high-risk neonate. *American Journal of Obstetrics and Gynecology, 117,* 1–9.

Holmes, D. L., Ruble, N., Kowalski, J., & Lauesen, B. (1984, March). *Predicting quality of attachment at one year from neonatal characteristics.* Paper presented at the International Conference on Infant Studies, New York.

Jeremy, R. J., & Bernstein, V. J. (1984). Dyads at risk: Methadone-maintained women and their four-month-old infants. *Child Development, 55,* 1141–1154.

Johnson, D., Krejci, C., Hack, M., & Fanaroff, A. (1984). Distribution of enamel defects and the association with respiratory distress in very low birthweight infants. *Journal of Dental Research, 63,* 59–64.

Jones, A. C. (1978). Life changes and psychological distress as predictors of pregnancy outcome. *Psychosomatic Medicine, 40,* 402–412.

Klusman, L. E. (1975). Reduction of pain in childbirth by the reduction of anxiety during pregnancy. *Journal of Consulting and Clinical Psychology, 43,* 162–165.

Koshland, D. (1987). Immortality and risk assessments. *Science, 236,* 241.

Kumar, R., & Robson, K. M. (1984). A prospective study of emotional disorders in childbearing women. *British Journal of Psychiatry, 144,* 35–47.

Lave, L. (1987). Health and safety risk analyses: Information for better decisions. *Science, 236,* 291–295.

Lederman, E., Lederman, R., Work, B., & McCann, D. (1981). Maternal psychological and physiologic correlates of fetal–newborn health status. *American Journal of Obstetrics and Gynecology, 139,* 956–958.

Lesinski, J. (1975). High-risk pregnancy. *Obstetrics and Gynecology, 46,* 599–603.

Lester, B., Emory, E., Hoffman, S., & Eitzman, D. (1976). A multivariate study of the effects of high risk factors on performance on the Brazelton Neonatal Assessment Scale. *Child Development, 47,* 515–517.

Lilford, R. J., & Chard, T. (1982). Computers in antenatal care. *British Journal of Hospital Medicine, 28,* 420–426.

Littman, B. (1980). In reply. *Pediatrics, 66,* 156.

Littman, B. & Parmelee, A. (1978). Medical correlation of infant development. *Pediatrics, 61,* 470–474.

Lubchenco, L. (1976). *The high risk infant.* Philadelphia: W. B. Saunders.

Lubchenco, L., Searls, D., & Brazie, J. (1972). Neonatal morbidity rate: Relationship to birthweight and gestational age. *Fetal and Neonatal Medicine, 81,* 814–822.

Lubin, B. (1965). Adjective checklist for measurement of depression. *Archives of General Psychiatry, 12,* 57–62.

Lunenfeld, I., Rosenthal, J., Larholt, K. M., & Insler, V. (1984). Childbirth experience—Psychological, cultural and medical associations. *Journal of Psychosomatic Obstetrics and Gynecology, 3,* 165–171.

Luz, N. P. (1985). Auditory evoked responses in the human fetus. *Acta Obstetrica et Gynecologica Scandinavia, 64,* 213–222.

Marcus, J., Auerback, J., Wilkinson, L., & Burack, C. M. (1981). Infants at risk for schizophrenia. *Archives of General Psychiatry, 38,* 703–713.

McDonald, R. L. (1968). The role of emotional factors in obstetric complications: A review. *Psychosomatic Medicine, 30,* 222–243.

McDonald, R. L., & Christakos, A. C. (1963). Relationship of emotional adjustment during pregnancy to obstetric complications. *American Journal of Obstetrics and Gynecology, 86,* 341–348.

McDonald, R. L., & Parham, K. (1964). Relation of emotional changes during pregnancy to obstetric complications in unmarried primigravidas. *American Journal of Obstetrics and Gynecology, 90,* 195–201.

Molfese, V. J., & Thomson, B. K. (1985). Optimality versus complications: Assessing predictive values of perinatal scales. *Child Development, 56,* 810–823.

Molfese, V. J., Thomson, B., & Bennett, A. (1985). Perinatal outcome: The similarity and predictive values of antepartum and intrapartum assessment scales. *Journal of Reproductive Medicine, 30,* 30–38.

Molfese, V., Thomson, B., Beadnell, B., Bricker, M. & Manion, L. (1987). Perinatal risk screening and infant outcome: Can predictions be improved with composite scales? *Journal of Reproductive Medicine, 32,* 569–576.

Molfese, V., Bricker, M., Manion, L., Beadnell, B., Yaple, K., & Moirs, K. (1987). Anxiety, depression and stress in pregnancy: A multivariate model of intrapartum risks and pregnancy outcome. *Journal of Psychosomatic Obstetrics and Gynecology, 7,* 77–92.

Molfese, V., Bricker, M., Manion, L., Yaple, K., & Beadnell, B. (1987). Stress in pregnancy: The influence of psychological and social mediators in perinatal experiences. *Journal of Psychosomatic Obstetrics and Gynecology, 6,* 33–42.

Morrison, I., Carter, L., McNamara, S., & Cheang, M. (1980). A simplified intrapartum numerical scoring system. *American Journal of Obstetrics and Gynecology, 138,* 175–181.

Morrison, I., & Olsen, J. (1979). Perinatal mortality and antepartum risk scoring. *Obstetrics and Gynecology, 53,* 362–366.

Munro, I. (1984). Pregnancy depression. *Lancet, 2,* 206.

Nesbitt, R., & Aubry, R. (1969). High-risk obstetrics. *American Journal of Obstetrics and Gynecology, 103,* 972–985.

Nesbitt, R., & Aubry, R. (1971). High-risk obstetrics IV: An evaluation of the effects of intensified care on pregnancy outcome. *American Journal of Obstetrics and Gynecology, 111,* 650–657.

Newton, R. W., & Hunt, L. P. (1984). Psychological stress in pregnancy and its relation to low birthweight. *British Medical Journal, 288,* 1191.

Niswander, K. R., & Gordon, M. (1972). *The Collaborative Perinatal Study of the National Institute of Neurological Diseases and Stroke. The Women and Their Pregnancies.* Philadelphia: W. B. Saunders.

Norbeck, J., & Tilden, V. (1983). Life stress, social support and emotional disequilibrium in complications of pregnancy: A prospective multivariate study. *Journal of Health and Social Behavior, 24,* 30–46.

Nuckolls, K., Cassel, J., & Kaplan, B. (1972). Psychological assets, life crises and the prognosis of pregnancy. *American Journal of Epidemiology, 95,* 431–441.

Obayuwana, A. O., Carter, A. L., & Barnett, R. M. (1984). Psychosocial distress and pregnancy outcome: A three-year prospective study. *Journal of Psychosomatic Obstetrics and Gynecology, 3,* 173–183.

O'Connell, M. (1983). Locus of control specific to pregnancy. *Journal of Obstretic Gynecology Nursing, 12,* 161–164.

O'Hara, M. W., Neunaber, O. J., & Zekoski, E. M. (1984). Prospective study of depression: Prevalence, course and predictive factors. *Journal of Abnormal Psychology, 93,* 158–171.

Parmelee, A., & Haber, A. (1973). Who is the "risk" infant? *Clinical Obstetrics and Gynecology, 16,* 376–387.

Parmelee, A., Kopp, C., & Sigman, M. (1976). Selection of development assessment techniques for infants at risk. *Merrill-Palmer Quarterly, 22,* 177–199.

Pilowsky, I., & Sharp, J. (1971). Psychological aspects of pre-eclamptic toxemia: A prospective study. *Journal of Psychosomatic Research, 15,* 193–197.

Powers, P. S., Johnson, T., Knuppel, R., Cupoli, J. M., & Achenback, K. E. (1986). Psychiatric disorders in high-risk pregnancy. *Comprehensive Psychiatry, 27,* 159–164.

Prechtl, H. F. R. (1967). Neurological sequelae of prenatal and perinatal complications. *British Medical Journal, 4,* 763–767.

Prechtl, H. F. R. (1968). Neurological findings in newborn infants after pre and paranatal complications. In J. Jonxis, H. Vissern, & J. Trodstran (Eds.), *Aspects of prematurity and dysmaturity: Nutricia Symposium* (pp. 305–321). Springfield, IL: Charles C Thomas.

Prechtl, H. F. R. (1981). Optimality: A new assessment concept. In C. Brown (Ed.), *Infants at risk: Assessment and intervention* (pp. 1–5). Skillman, NJ: Johnson & Johnson.

Prechtl, H. F. R., & Beintema, D. (1964). *The neurological examination of the full-term newborn infant.* Little Club Clinics in Developmental Medicine (No. 12). Philadelphia: Lippincott.

Rees, W., & Lutkins, S. (1971). Parental depression before and after childbirth. *Journal of the Royal College of General Practitioners, 21,* 26–31.

Reich, J. W., Holmes, D. L., Slaymaker, F. L., Lauesen, B. F., & Gyurke, J. S. (1984, March). *Infant assessments as predictors of 3-year IQ.* Paper presented at the International Conference on Infant Studies, New York.

Remo, H., Largo, D., Pfister, G. (1987, April). *Significance of pre-, peri-, and post-natal events for language, cognitive, and neurological development in preterm children aged 5–7 years.* Paper presented at the meeting of the Society for Research in Child Development, Baltimore.

Rishpon, S., Epstein, L. M., & Egoz, N. (1985). Association of infant mortality with lack of regular prenatal care in the Haifa Subdistrict, 1980. *Israel Journal of Medical Sciences, 21,* 123–126.

Rizzardo, I., Magni, G., Andreoli, C., Merlin, G., Andreoli, F., Cosentino, M., & Ziglio, R. (1982). Life events and obstetric complications: A preliminary report. *Psychological Reports, 51,* 1035–1038.

Rose, S., Schmidt, K., Riese, M., & Bridges, W. (1980). Effects of prematurity and early intervention on responsivity to tactual stimuli: A comparison of preterm and full-term infants. *Child Development, 51,* 416–425.

Rosenberg, S. N., Albertsen, P. C., Jones, E. E., & Roberts, R. S. (1981). Complications of labor and delivery following uncomplicated pregnancy. *Medical Care, 19,* 68–79.

Rosengren, W. R. (1961). Some social psychological aspects of delivery room difficulties. *Journal of Nervous and Mental Disorders, 132,* 515–521.

Rotter, J., Chance, J., & Phares, E. (1972). *Applications of a social learning theory of personality.* New York: Holt, Rinehart & Winston.

Roux, J. F. (1976). Labor monitoring and fetal health. *Obstetrics and Gynecology Annual, 5,* 139–165.

Ryan, G., Sweeney, P., & Solola, A. (1980). Pregnancy care and pregnancy outcome. *American Journal of Obstetrics and Gynecology, 137,* 876–881.

Salter, M., Holmes, D., Reich, J., & Slaymaker, F. (1987). *The relation of maternal attitudes and expectations to later perceptions of infants.* Unpublished doctoral dissertation, Loyola University of Chicago.

Sameroff, A. (1979). The etiology of creative competence: A systems perspective. In R. Kearsley & I. Siegal (Eds.), *Infants at risk: Assessment of cognitive functioning* (pp. 115–151). New York: Wiley.

Sameroff, A., & Chandler, M. (1975). Reproductive risk and the continuum of caretaking casualty. In F. D. Horowitz (Ed.), *Review of child development research* (Vol. 4). Chicago: University of Chicago Press.

Sameroff, A., Seifer, R., & Zax, M. (1982). Early development of children at risk for emotional disorder. *Monographs of the Society for Research in Child Development, 47* (1, Serial No. 199).

Sarason, T. G. (1979). *Life stress, self-preoccupation, and social supports* (Technical Report No. SCS-LS-008, Office of Naval Research). Washington, DC: U.S. Government Printing Office.

Seifer, R., Sameroff, A., & Jones, F. (1981). Adaptive behavior in young children of emotionally disturbed women. *Journal of Applied Developmental Psychology, 1,* 251–276.

Sepkoski, C., Coll, C., & Lester, B. (1977, March). *The effects of high risk factors on neonatal behavior as measured by the Brazelton scale.* Paper presented at the meeting of the Society for Research in Child Development, New Orleans.

Sepkoski, C., Coll, C., & Lester, B. (1982). The cumulative effects of obstetric risk variables on newborn behavior. In L. Lipsitt & T. Field (Eds.), *Infant behavior and development: Perinatal risk and newborn behavior* (pp. 33–39). Norwood, NJ: Ablex.

Shapiro, S., Schlesinger, E. R., & Nesbitt, R. E. L., Jr. (1968). *Infant, perinatal, maternal, and childhood mortality in the United States.* Cambridge, MA: Harvard University Press.

Shaw, J., Wheeler, P., & Morgan, M. (1970). Emotions during pregnancy. *Journal of the American Child Psychiatrist, 9,* 428–444.

Simmons, F. B. (1978). Identification of hearing loss in infants and young children. *Otolaryngologic Clinics of North America, 11,* 55–61.

Smilkste, G. (1984). Prediction of pregnancy complications: An application of the biopsychological model. *Social Sciences and Medicine, 18,* 315.

Sokol, R. J., Rosen, M. G., Stojkov, J., & Chik, L. (1977). Clinical application of high-risk scoring on an obstetric service. *American Journal of Obstetrics and Gynecology, 128,* 652–661.

Sokol, R. J., Woolf, R., Rosen, M., & Weingarden, K. (1980). Risk, antenatal care, and outcome: Impact of a maternity infant care project. *Obstetrics and Gynecology, 58,* 150–156.

Spielberger, C. D., Gorsuch, R. L., & Luschene, R. E. (1970). *STAI manual.* Palo Alto, CA: Consulting Psychologists Press.

Stanley, K., Soule, B., & Copans, S. A. (1979). Dimensions of prenatal anxiety and their influence on pregnancy outcome. *American Journal of Obstetrics and Gynecology, 135,* 22–26.

Strobino, D. M., & Baruffi, G. (1984). Evaluation of a measure of neonatal morbidity. *Medical Care, 22,* 818–826.

Sylvain, J. P. E. (1984). Regionalization of perinatal services and the use of high-risk scoring forms. *Canadian Medical Association Journal, 130,* 1269–1271.

Tilden, V. (1983). The relation of life stress and social support to emotional disequilibrium during pregnancy. *Research Nursing Health, 6,* 167–174.

Unter, C. E. M. (1982). Waikato Women's Hospital newborn transit service: The first year's experience. *New Zealand Medical Journal, 95,* 683–688.

Vaux, A. (1982). *Measure of three levels of social support: Resources, behaviors, and feelings.* Unpublished manuscript. (Available from the author, Department of Psychology, Southern Illinois University, Carbondale, IL 62901.)

Warheit, G. J. (1979). Life events, coping, stress and depressive symtomatology. *American Journal of Psychiatry, 136,* 502–507.

Watson, J., Elliott, S., Rugg, A., & Borough, D. (1984). Psychiatric disorder in pregnancy and the first postnatal year. *British Journal of Psychiatry, 144,* 453–462.

Werner, J., Bartlett, A., & Siqueland E. (1982). Assessment of preterm and full-term infants. In L. Lipsett & T. Fields (Eds.), *Infant behavior and development: Perinatal risk and newborn behavior* (pp. 131–138). Norwood, NJ: Ablex

Widmayer, S. M., & Field, T. M. (1980). Effects of Brazelton demonstrations on early interactions of preterm infants and their teenage mothers. *Infant Behavior and Development, 3,* 79–89.

Williams, C. C., Williams, R. A., Griswold, M. J., & Holmes, T. H. (1975). Pregnancy and life change. *Journal of Psychosomatic Research, 19,* 123–129.

Wilson, R., & Crouch, E. (1987). Risk assessment and comparisons: An introduction. *Science, 236,* 267–270.

Wilson, R. W., & Schifrin, B. S. (1980). Ideas & actions: Is any pregnancy low risk? *Obstetrics and Gynecology, 55,* 653–661.

Woodson, R. (1987, April). *Neonatal behavior: Unreliable yet careful.* Paper presented at the meeting of the Society for Research in Child Development, Baltimore.

Wrate, R. M., Rooney, A. C., Thomas, P. F., & Cox, J. L. (1985). Postnatal depression and child development: A three-year follow-up study. *British Journal of Psychiatry, 146,* 622–627.

Yamamoto, K. J., & Kinney, D. K. (1976). Pregnant women's ratings of different factors influencing psychological stress during pregnancy. *Psychological Reports, 39,* 203–214.

Zajicek, E., & Wolkind, S. (1978). Emotional difficulties in married women during and after the first pregnancy. *British Journal of Medical Psychology, 51,* 379–385.

Zax, M., Sameroff, A. J., & Babigian, H. M. (1977). Birth outcomes in the offspring of mentally disordered women. *American Journal of Orthopsychiatry, 47,* 218–230.

Zax, M., Sameroff, A. J., & Farnum, A. J. (1975). Childbirth education, marital attitudes, and delivery. *American Journal of Obstetrics and Gynecology, 123,* 185–190.

Zeskind, P. S., & Iacinco, R. (1984). Effects of maternal visitation to preterm infants in the neonatal intensive care unit. *Child Development, 55,* 1887–1893.

Zuckerman, M., Nurnberger, J. I., Gardiner, S. H., Vandiveer, J. M., Barrett, B. H., & Denbreeijen, A. (1963). Psychological correlates of somatic complaints in pregnancy and difficulty in childbirth. *Journal of Consulting Psychology, 27,* 324–329.

Index

G

H

I

R

S